FITTER, HAPPIER

RHETORIC, CULTURE, AND SOCIAL CRITIQUE

FITTER, HAPPIER

The Eugenic Strain in Twentieth-Century Cancer Rhetoric

LOIS PETERS AGNEW

THE UNIVERSITY OF ALABAMA PRESS
Tuscaloosa

The University of Alabama Press
Tuscaloosa, Alabama 35487-0380
uapress.ua.edu

Typeface: Arno Pro

Cover image: Paul Bragg and hikers, Hollywood Hills, Los Angeles, ca. 1930, photo CL Whitt (0778); "Dick" Whittington Studio Collection of Negatives and Photographs, the Huntington Library, San Marino, California.

Cover design: Sandy Turner Jr.

Cataloging-in-Publication data is available from the Library of Congress.
ISBN: 978-0-8173-2185-7 (cloth)
ISBN: 978-0-8173-6134-1 (paper)
E-ISBN: 978-0-8173-9487-5

FOR MY PARENTS, WHOSE RESPONSE TO CANCER EMBODIED GRACE AND COURAGE THAT CANNOT BE CAPTURED BY METAPHOR, AND FOR PETE, ELIZABETH, PETER, MIKE, LUKE, AND CALEB, WHOSE LOVE, STRENGTH, AND JOY ANIMATE ALL MY WORK.

CONTENTS

PREFACE

Events in my life have made me well aware of the ubiquity of cancer and of the reasons people are so afraid of it. My father began a long journey with cancer when I was twelve years old, my mother developed stage four ovarian cancer twelve years after his death, and both my husband and sister were diagnosed with chronic lymphocytic leukemia more than a decade ago. During my work on revising this manuscript, my daughter was diagnosed with lymphoma of the skin, which was something I'd never heard of. And across the years I have seen many friends go through the ups and downs of cancer treatment and experience varying degrees of success in their pursuit of full recovery. In the midst of these experiences of seeing cancer's effects on the people I love, I have noticed how distant the common ways of talking about cancer are from the daily experiences people have with the disease. Even from a young age, I couldn't help wondering where these rhetorical stragegies came from and why they had achieved such prominence and staying power when they didn't seem particularly useful.

My academic training in rhetorical studies has provided me with frameworks for thinking about these questions, as well as more complicated ways of conceiving of questions pertaining to why particular lines of argument have such staying power. As the daughter, sister, wife, and mother of cancer patients, I might interpret lines of argument about cancer as worthless, but when I looked at these arguments through the lens of my professional training in rhetorical studies, I was forced to look more deeply at the cultural purposes served by topoi that have evolved and persisted across an entire century. This perspective led me to shift from my original question, "Why do these arguments still exist?" to ask, "For whom do these arguments exist, and what purpose do they serve?"

My research in rhetorical history provided me with an avenue for beginning to investigate some of the starting points for what I identified as significant cancer topoi: dominant lines of argument about cancer that have circulated across decades of the twentieth century. My investigation of these topoi led me to several archives, along with primary sources written by people with cancer and secondary sources about cancer history. What I have produced is not a medical history but a rhetorical history focused on prominent lines of argument about cancer. These lines of argument do not function in a linear manner; the chapters in this book therefore cannot be neatly divided into discrete time periods defined by the rise of a specific topos. Instead, each chapter focuses on a topos that developed in response to the strategic decision to publicize cancer that took place early in the twentieth century and then traces the ways in which that topos continues to circulate in ways that reflect and further shape cultural perspectives across subsequent decades in that century.

My academic interest in disability studies provided me with further insight about the power of cancer topoi focused on mounting a strong, determined, and intelligent response to cancer. The "overcoming" narrative imposed on people with disabilities applies in a slightly different way to people with cancer. Certainly, cancer patients and their families crave reassurance following the terror of a cancer diagnosis. However, the suggestion that cancer can be managed through sheer force of will exerted by people with cancer does not truly provide reassurance for those individuals, because their daily experience tells them that the situation is not so simple. But the insistence that cancer can be defeated through the efforts of people who are unfortunate enough to become ill has never been primarily directed toward the needs of cancer patients but has arisen from a long-standing determination to turn away from weakness, to maintain the illusion that American strength and ingenuity can solve every human problem.

The urgent quest for perfection accounts for the prominence of eugenic ideologies early in the twentieth century, but it is important to recognize that this perspective has by no means disappeared decades later. This is evident because cancer topoi continue to be important in the present day in ways that are not accounted for in my archival sources. However, it is my hope that a focused view of these rhetorical conceptions of the ideal response to cancer, the people who are constructed through these frameworks, and the cultural values and assumptions that they support can provide a foundation for future interrogation of the complicated relationship between language, public health, and the pursuit of an elusive norm that has played such a prominent role in the US social imagination.

ACKNOWLEDGMENTS

I am deeply grateful for all of the support I've received in working on this project. The archival materials used in this manuscript are courtesy of: the Memorial Sloan Kettering Cancer Center Library and Archives, housed in the Rockefeller Archive Center, Sleepy Hollow, New York; the Lasker Foundation, which gave me permission to use their materials housed in the Rare Book and Manuscript Library at Columbia University in the City of New York; Rare Books and Early Manuscripts, History of Medicine Division, US National Library of Medicine; and the Historical Resources Center, Research Medical Library, the University of Texas MD Anderson Cancer Center.

I would also like to give special thanks to the archivists and staff members who supported my research and preparations for publication: Kathleen Brennan and Sheridan Sayles with the MSKCC Library and Archives; Jose Javier Garza with the Historical Resources Center, Research Medical Library, at the University of Texas MD Anderson Cancer Center; Courtney Nandagiri, administrative and program manager at the Lasker Foundation; and Stephen J. Greenberg, section head for rare books and early manuscripts in the History of Medicine Division at the National Library of Medicine. I'm also grateful to Lauren Esposito for providing research assistance early in the project. I am grateful to Syracuse University for the generous research support that supported my travel to conduct archival research and for the intellectual environment that has stimulated my thinking about this project. I'm also grateful to Daniel Waterman, editor in chief of the University of Alabama Press, for his remarkable support and patience in guiding me through this process and for the helpful guidance from the anonymous readers. Finally, special thanks to my husband, Pete, who helped me with the conception for this project and has supported me in so many ways during my work.

This book is derived in part from an article published in *Rhetoric Society Quarterly* 50, no. 3 (2020): 194–202, copyright Rhetoric Society of America, available online, and an article published in *College English* 80, no. 3 (2018): 271–96, published by the National Council of Teachers of English.

FITTER, HAPPIER

Introduction

US Cancer Rhetoric

CONSTRUCTING A PEOPLE

After exercising supreme caution to protect my immunocompromised family member during the early months of the pandemic, access to the COVID-19 vaccine and declining case numbers in the summer of 2021 made me bold enough to stand in line at a local restaurant to pick up my family's first take-out meal since the spring of 2020. Most patrons wore masks as I did, but the man who took his place behind me in line not only chose not to wear a mask but also complained loudly about all of us who had chosen to do so. I stood there shocked as he launched a wide array of expletives denouncing the "Democrats" who were so concerned about an illness he had chosen not to think about. I was horrified by his hostility and baffled by his apparent politicization of public health. But given my interest in rhetorics of health and medicine, I should not have been so surprised. As this book will show, risks frequently come from the act of making vulnerability visible. A major challenge facing those who care about public health lies in the need to make people aware of issues that they would prefer not to think about.

This tension has defined the development of cancer rhetorics since the early decades of the twentieth century. During that period, the concerted effort to make people aware of cancer as a prominent public health concern was consistently undermined by a strong cultural emphasis on strength, autonomy, and social progress. Although cancer has obvious differences from contagious illnesses such as COVID-19, many of the cultural values at work in public arguments about the pandemic also underlie lines of argument about cancer that emerged and flourished in the early decades of the twentieth century. They also reflect the difficult balance between making visible the effects of illness on individuals and outlining the steps required in a general response to public health concerns. In *Governing Systems: Modernity and the Making of Public Health in England, 1830–1910,* Tom Crook describes the development of modern public health systems as situated in a shift from localized support structures to those operating at "central and international levels,"[1] a transformation that is strikingly evident in the early twentieth-century rise of national centers specializing in cancer research and treatment. At the same time, Crook argues that this transition functions alongside "a reinvigoration of the local and the personal."[2] While modernization assigns power to professionals and experts, it is based simultaneously in a democratic impulse that provides individuals with agency and opportunities for self-governance, including asserting control over decisions pertaining to their health. Thus, for Crook, modern medicine is defined by a "process of mutual elaboration and transformation" that includes a dynamic interaction between personal decision-making and the conglomeration of expertise needed to advance scientific progress and the welfare of the collective.[3]

This dynamic takes on a particular tenor in US public health rhetorics, where the need to pursue collective interests comes up against a national ethos grounded in tough-minded individualism. The view that everyone benefits from the success of individuals has historically been complicated by the assumption that those individuals' contributions to the collective good can best be achieved through the embodiment of culturally endorsed qualities that sustain the expected norm, which has excluded from consideration the wide range of individual identities, aptitudes, and health conditions that can be found across the population. Thus, US public health has often been conceived in terms of those who fulfill the image of the American ideal through strength, self-sufficiency, and resilience and therefore prove that good health is readily accessible without dependence on others.

US rhetorics of public health both illustrate and complicate the rhetorical process of forming a people as described by Michael McGee in his landmark essay "In Search of 'The People': A Rhetorical Alternative." McGee argues that "the people" do not objectively exist but are constantly under construction through rhetoric: "In purely objective terms, the only human reality is that of the individual; groups, whether as small as a Sunday School class or as big as a whole society, are infused with an artificial identity. So from a rhetorical perspective, the entire socialization process is nothing but intensive and continual exercises in persuasion: Individuals must be seduced into abandoning their individuality, convinced of their sociality."[4] Rhetorics of public health are signal examples of a process in which the intensity of individual experiences with disease are subsumed by the need to identify generalizable risks and prescribe desirable behaviors and treatments that apply to "the public," a challenging enterprise in a society in which individuals are conditioned against those seductive forces that might sway them toward "abandoning their individuality." The complexity of this interplay in US public health discourses frequently generates rhetorical strategies that assure people that their participation in the larger group will hold benefits without requiring that they give up the individual privileges they hold dear. In the case of cancer rhetoric, the focus on public health concerns against the backdrop of a strong cultural emphasis on individual strength and resilience generates lines of argument that construct not so much a true collective "people" but a loosely connected group of individuals whose discipline, disposition, and intelligence can protect them from the most disabling effects of disease, even as most people who have cancer are likely to have a very different kind of experience.

This book traces the way in which lines of argument about cancer form such a "people," a group united by a shared concern about the threat of cancer but whose collective identity is also defined by an outlook that assures them of their ability to maintain comfortable distance from the complex experiences of individuals with cancer. Drawing from a range of archival materials, I argue that the cultural contexts surrounding twentieth-century US cancer rhetoric contribute to the construction of "a people" that embodies larger value systems that include self-sufficiency, resilience, and strength of will. This alignment reflects an ongoing tension in public health rhetorics, as the public created by cancer rhetoric must acknowledge the threat the disease poses to the well-being of the collective but at the same time persistently leaves responsibility for managing the threat not only in the hands of medical researchers but also implicitly in the hands of individuals who contribute to the public's well-being through personal qualities that will help them overcome the most devastating effects of disease. There is little doubt that cancer patients are unable to achieve the ideal that is rhetorically constructed through these lines of argument; however, their rhetorical function resides not in capturing the experiences of people who are ill but in sustaining the deeply entrenched American image of personal autonomy, economic strength, and modern progress.

The rhetorical history that follows examines publicly circulated arguments about cancer that emerged with the strategic deployment of publicity about cancer as a health threat in the early twentieth century, with a focus on three dominant topoi, central lines of argument that people return to repeatedly in order to develop particular interpretations of human experience that are sustained across several decades. This book does not offer a comprehensive history of medical developments in cancer research and treatment; instead, it focuses on prominent lines of argument that illustrate the challenges associated with making cancer visible in an environment in which the need for confidence in American strength and self-sufficiency was so powerful. The circulation of cancer publicity in the early twentieth century draws together a complex network of ideas, as the urgency of communicating about cancer as a threat to public health simultaneously created "a people" poised to respond to that threat. Each of the dominant cancer topoi crystallizes for an anxious public the idealized qualities that can achieve this goal: strong and determined against the enemy, capable of maintaining a positive outlook that will miraculously overcome the effects of cancer, and equipped to protect themselves against cancer through vigilance and intelligence. These topoi are embedded in larger cultural contexts that include scientific advances in cancer research as well as cultural logics that define appropriate responses to public health crises and in the process suppress unmanageable alternatives. Cancer topoi therefore constitute rhetorical frameworks that emerge from what McGee refers to as "dormant arguments," which, as he explains, "do not define 'the people' at a specific moment, but they do represent the parameters of what 'the people' of that culture could possibly become."[5] The project of determining what the American ideal of self-sufficient strength can become in the face of an uncontrollable adversary yields cancer topoi that engage with dynamic medical developments while working within and shaping the parameters of established cultural prescriptions for "what 'the people' of that culture could possibly become."[6]

CANCER AND RHETORIC: THE MANY SIDES OF PUBLICITY

The fear of cancer is not a twentieth-century phenomenon, as the view of this disease as a mysterious and deadly health menace has existed since ancient times. While the primal dread of cancer as a threat to life was sustained through the twentieth century, evolving lines of argument during this period reflect a shift in the way cancer is represented. This shift begins with the strategic decision to bring cancer into public view for the first time. Prior to the twentieth century, cancer was a private matter that was rarely mentioned in public, based on the notions that the disease was somehow shameful and that families were best equipped to handle hopeless illness, as well as disability, internally. One effect of this approach was that society was protected from the need to encounter undesirable problems pertaining to bodies and health. Sharon L. Snyder and David T. Mitchell explain that the "tradition of treating disability as a private family matter functioned as a form of social invisibility," a quality that also extended to cancer.[7]

This point underscores the fact that silence is itself a rhetorical choice; as Cheryl Glenn has pointed out, speech and silence "are inextricably linked and often interchangeably, simultaneously meaningful."[8] Viewed through this lens, we can see that cancer rhetoric did exist before the twentieth century, as cancer, the identity of patients, and the appropriate public response were constructed through that which could not be spoken as well as through twentieth-century lines of argument that instructed people about cancer and persuaded them to take action. For this reason, my argument is not that cancer rhetoric originates in the twentieth century, but instead that the recognition of cancer as a matter for public concern during that time period led to a transition from silence and privacy to public arguments aimed at creating a people prepared to take an active role in limiting the disease's threat to public health.

The strategic decision to use persuasive measures to inform and move the public is an important part of the history of cancer. While medical discoveries advance through scientific processes that are somewhat distinct from the realm of public rhetoric, Judy Segal points out that rhetoric plays a crucial role in that "discourse fills the space that certainty in medicine leaves unoccupied."[9] The attempt to come to terms with the medical uncertainty surrounding cancer accounts for the power of cancer topoi, commonplaces that people return to repeatedly to generate familiar arguments that assert a measure of collective control over the disease, a significant value during a period in which the modern goals of progress, order, and control were prominent. A number of the characteristic features of cancer, including its ubiquity, unpredictability, and resilience, have yielded commonplace arguments that circulate across public, private, and medical contexts. These arguments collectively serve the explicit goal of educating the public about the latest medical knowledge available, but they also manage the anxiety created by this knowledge through supporting the formation of a public confident that cancer can be partially controlled as individuals cultivate particular behaviors and dispositions, even if a medical cure is not yet on the horizon.

The tension between the need to acknowledge the real danger of cancer and the American insistence upon confidence and control lies at the heart of cancer rhetoric. Lines of argument that draw attention to the threat of cancer simultaneously require assurance that cancer, like all other dangers, can be conquered through the unique American qualities of strength, self-sufficiency, intelligence, and progress. The conflicting impulses in cancer rhetoric reflect larger cultural patterns of suppressing differences as soon as they become visible. In their discussion of Henri-Jacques Stiker's history of disability, Snyder and Mitchell write, "It is as if a deviance in the accepted order of things implies that society must master difference in order to turn aside an omen of things to come."[10] Because cancer publicity demands an acknowledgment of cancer as a public danger, drawing attention to "a deviance in the accepted order of things," it simultaneously requires lines of argument that offer evidence of society's ability to "master difference."[11] The people constructed through cancer rhetoric therefore illustrate McGee's assertion that "the people" inevitably "exist in objective reality and as social fantasies at the same time,"[12] as cancer rhetoric transforms the physical realities of geographical location, disease, and vulnerability into the fantasy of a people prepared to adopt actions and attitudes that enact a national destiny to overcome disease through strength of will. Cancer rhetoric can tell us much about the assumptions that govern how cancer research is represented to an anxious public, the evolution in public attitudes toward disease, and the lived experiences of people whose identities, outlooks, and, at times, decisions are shaped not only by the effects of their disease but also by language that defines appropriate responses to illness.

CANCER, RHETORIC, AND DISABILITY

The impulse to use rhetoric to construct a people capable of overcoming the effects of cancer creates an alignment between cancer and disability. Although disability is in many respects distinct from a chronic illness such as cancer, the lens of disability studies can be helpful in understanding how cancer rhetoric establishes a pattern of normative responses to the phenomenon of disease and why those normative responses are so compelling. At the same time, to assert a connection between cancer and disability rhetoric is a fraught enterprise in light of the problematic historical relationship between medicine and disability. As many disability studies scholars have demonstrated, the "medical model" assumes that disability is an objective physical reality that can best be addressed through medical intervention that potentially restores individuals to a more "normal" state, rather than through an examination of the social conditions that have constituted and imposed the ideal of normality in the first place. In addition to this fundamental concern, Susan Wendell notes that the medicalization of disability has contributed to the assumption that people with disabilities are "globally incapacitated" and that the best quality of life available for people with disabilities comes about through institutionalization.[13] She posits impairment as a category that merits greater attention both within and beyond the disability community, as it acknowledges the distinction between disability and illness while offering insight into the ways in which both disability and chronic illness benefit from careful exploration of social structures that function to marginalize members of both communities.

In drawing from disability scholarship to inform the analysis of cancer rhetoric, I am building on Wendell's view of the benefits inherent in recognizing parallels between the experiences of those who deal with impaired health and people with disabilities, even as it is critical that we never lose sight of the differences in their situations. In *A History of Disability*, Henri-Jacques Stiker notes that the connection between disease and death leads to a divergence between illness and "the fear of the abnormal" that pervades disability.[14] However, Stiker acknowledges that "the dividing line is not always sharp," adding that "disease, death, and monstrosity certainly come together at one point: in the desire to kill. We should not hide from the fact that major disability, especially mental, generates such an urge to make it disappear that it might be called by its name."[15] While the desire to kill is not directed toward people with cancer, the explicit goal of cancer's disappearance often entails the less obvious impulse to make the uncomfortable experiences of people with cancer disappear as well. This insight acknowledges the tensions characteristic of the public dissemination of cancer rhetoric, which directly engages with what Annemarie Mol describes as the distinction between disease, "the object of biomedicine," and the culturally sanctioned response to illness that determines "a patient's interpretation of his or her disease, the feelings that accompany it, the life event it turns into."[16]

The life event of disease occurs in ways that are both pervasive and particular to individual circumstances, a feature that cancer rhetorics often obliterate through constructing a public aware of its vulnerability to cancer but at the same time determined to assert the capacity of individuals to overcome its most devastating effects. Despite the variable nature of cancer and disability, the connections between disability and diseases such as cancer are evident in the complex discursive and material structures that promote awareness and overcoming, make bodies visible and invisible, and encourage people to gaze upon images of disease and disability as a public health problem to be solved, without fully attending to the human experiences of those who inhabit disabled and diseased bodies. As is the case with disability, individuals' experiences with cancer are not only physical phenomena but are also socially and rhetorically constructed. Lynda Birke argues that "people with diseases, or some forms of physical disability, may well experience their bodily interiors differently from persons who are well or able-bodied: but part of that experience depends upon the cultural experience of living out medical definitions of pathological functioning."[17] A. Suresh Canagarajah describes his own journey with the disabling effects of disease following his cancer diagnosis: "My status as disabled was socially constructed. There were long-standing social discourses that informed the attitudes of my acquaintances, relatives, and physicians. Their conversations reflected biases relating to fundamental definitions on what it means to be able, normal, and human."[18] Both cancer patients and people with disabilities deviate from what Rosemarie Garland-Thomson has described as the "normate," the assumed standard that imagines an identity free from the stigma associated with characteristics that depart from those valued by the surrounding culture.[19] The twentieth-century formation of cancer rhetoric in the United States simultaneously acknowledges cancer as a public health concern and develops topoi that subsume individual experiences within normalized responses that reinscribe the values of strength and self-sufficiency while circumventing possibilities that fail to align with those values.

CANCER, DISABILITY, AND EUGENICS

The strong cultural urge to create a world based on normalcy and progress affects both people with disabilities and those with chronic diseases such as cancer. And it is this urge that accounts for the prominence of eugenic ideologies, which emerged in the early twentieth century in concert with a growing preoccupation with modern goals of productivity, strength, and scientific and industrial progress. In some respects, it might seem surprising to connect cancer with disability in the first place, and a further step is required to make a connection between cancer and eugenic ideologies. Eugenics is generally understood to be a program that pursued social improvement through purifying the race of inferior genetic strains, most often through scientific endeavors such as testing, breeding, and sterilization programs. At first glance, the entirely positive goal of eradicating a life-threatening disease such as cancer appears to have little to do with the problematic methods and objectives associated with eugenics.

Delving more deeply into the underlying assumptions and motives that surrounded eugenics presents a more complicated picture. First of all, there are some direct links between early cancer research and eugenics. For example, Clarence Cook Little, a prominent figure in cancer research through his role as managing director of the American Society for the Control of Cancer from 1929 to 1945 and director of the Jackson Laboratory at Cold Spring Harbor, also served as director of the American Eugenics Society from 1923 to 1939 and president of the organization in 1929. Furthermore, geneticist Kat Arney argues that early insights about the relationship between cancer and genetics were used by eugenicists dedicated to the goal of protecting society from "defective strains."[20] And in fact eugenic arguments were often entwined with early genetic research, as eugenicists considered the goal of protecting society from mental and physical disabilities and diseases to be a logical outcome of research into the genetic causes of these imperfections. In a 1921 address at the Second International Congress of Eugenics, Henry Fairfield Osborne argued, "As science has enlightened government in the prevention and spread of disease, it must also enlighten government in the spread and multiplication of worthless members of society, the spread of feeblemindedness, of idiocy, and of all moral and intellectual as well as physical diseases."[21] While cancer was not the primary target for eugenic intervention, research that sought to identify the genetic causes of cancer was not entirely protected from those who sought to draw from that research to support the goal of purifying society from the threat of all potential sources of debilitating genetic influences.

While evidence points toward some direct connections between certain lines of cancer research and eugenics, the focus of my argument is neither to prove that those connections exist nor to suggest that any direct connections account for the presence of eugenic strains in cancer rhetoric. However, I will argue that it is always the case that rhetoric reflects the culture that surrounds it, and cancer rhetoric is no exception. Eugenic ideologies were highly influential in the United States during the 1920s and 1930s, which coincides with the growing prominence of cancer research centers. The same period also saw the formation of cancer advocacy groups dedicated to the cause of bringing cancer into the public view, and many of these groups were connected with a scientific community that was in varying degrees influenced by eugenic thought. I am interested in tracing the presence of these influences, which entails exploring how prominent lines of argument about cancer implicitly advance the eugenic emphasis on progress, strength, and racial betterment that had such a powerful influence on US intellectual and cultural life during the early decades of the twentieth century.

In the introduction to *Popular Eugenics: National Efficiency and Mass Culture in the 1930s,* Susan Currell and Christine Cogdell describe the 1930s as a decade in which "educational and scientific discourses were permeated with eugenic rhetoric."[22] Eugenics can be seen as central to the constellation of ideas around which the rejection of difference has evolved, an insight reflected in Jay Dolmage's definition of eugenics as "the 'science' of controlling who lives, who procreates, who thrives, and who dies, based on flawed ideas about our genetic makeup."[23] Dolmage also emphasizes the dominance of this philosophy, noting that "beginning at the turn of the twentieth century, eugenics characterized and drove North American national health and immigration policy."[24] Snyder and Mitchell further discuss the widespread dissemination of eugenic thought within the medical community and across American society, countering the widespread view that eugenics was "a momentary aberration in the history of disability science" and arguing that with this view "we risk forgetting or diminishing widespread professional participation in a disgraceful historical chapter."[25] Part of the task of recognizing the ubiquity of eugenics in American social life has entailed a change in perspective; Wendy Kline notes that scholars in the 1990s shifted from focusing on eugenics as a science-based initiative toward recognizing its presence as a social movement: "Scholars discovered that eugenic ideology and social programs affected earlier Americans at multiple levels—from the fiction they read, to the movies they viewed, to the biology textbooks they learned from, to the exhibits they viewed at county fairs."[26]

The broad endorsement of eugenics and the prominence of eugenic thought in many areas of public life in the United States is indeed a shocking commentary on the national attitude toward people with disabilities, but the ubiquity of eugenic thought over a long period of time also makes it difficult to pinpoint the guiding principles of this national orientation or to narrow its goals of promoting the social, economic, racial, physical, and intellectual perfection of the nation. As Paul A. Lombardo notes, eugenics was both a set of ideas popular with the American public and a collection of goals and practices that were ever shifting: "The rationales that lawmakers and other officials voiced in support of 'eugenic' practices were clothed in ideas that had popular resonance. What 'eugenics' meant for the seven decades it was imbedded in U.S. law depended on what other ideas were used to justify it. Those ideas could include hereditary degeneracy, social and economic efficiency, neo-Malthusian population policy, or 'sins of the father' religious determinism."[27] He adds that to understand eugenics requires historical sensitivity, for "context is critical; both the idea of eugenics and the practices it led to had many faces."[28]

The faces of eugenics coalesce in the entrenchment of values that include modern progress, strength, self-sufficiency, and a stalwart commitment to "the normal." Douglas C. Baynton traces the modern focus on normality to the mid-nineteenth century, an emphasis that emerged "in the context of a pervasive belief in progress."[29] According to Baynton, the ideal of normality corresponded with the emergence of an evolutionary vision of society, replacing the earlier emphasis on "the natural" that prior to that time had been part of "what was seen as an essentially unchanging world."[30] Baynton goes on to explain, "Just as the counterpart to the natural was the monstrous, so the opposite of the normal person was the defective. Although normality ostensibly denoted the average, the usual, and the ordinary, in actual usage it functioned as an ideal and excluded only those defined as *below* average."[31] The transition from the natural to the normal places chronic illness within the scope of eugenics. An illness such as cancer might be seen as a natural part of human life, particularly as it originates in the body's own cells, but it constitutes an abnormality in those cells that not only represents a threat to the health of the individual but also illustrates the unpredictable corruption of normality and underscores the vulnerability that lies just below the surface of society's fervent hopes for ultimate progress toward perfection. While early cancer researchers made clear the challenges of determining how the genetic abnormality of cancer could be reversed, cancer topoi offered normalizing responses to a condition that was anything but normal.

CANCER, EUGENICS, AND ECONOMICS

The eugenic pursuit of "economic self-sufficiency" has important implications for public health rhetorics from the 1920s forward.[32] As has been the case during the COVID-19 pandemic, an important feature of the normalizing impulse characteristic of US cancer and disability rhetorics is based on economic concerns. Strength and self-sufficiency have been central values throughout US history; the evolution of capitalism in the twentieth century increasingly linked these values to the perceived economic well-being of the nation. Nirmala Erevelles's claim that "the human body is one of the most fetishized commodities in late-capitalist societies" offers useful insight for an analysis of both cancer and disability rhetorics, as neither of these embodied differences fit the ideal considered to be a crucial component of the nation's economic power.[33] Iris Marion Young highlights this point in describing the assumed ideal worker: "The 'normal' worker is supposed to be energetic, have high concentration abilities, be alert to adapt to changing conditions, and be able to withstand the physical, mental or interactive stress in good humor. Workers who fail to measure up to one or more of these standards are 'normally' considered lazy, slackers, uncooperative or otherwise inadequate. All workers must worry about *failing* in the eyes of their employers."[34] The threat of this failure became increasingly pronounced through the ascendancy of neoliberalism, which creates what Henry Giroux describes as "hyper-market-driven societies [that] organized identities largely as consumers."[35] Lennard Davis's reflections on the social function of normalcy offer a useful lens for understanding cancer rhetoric and its evolution across decades of the twentieth century: "The idea of a norm is less a condition of human nature than it is a feature of a certain kind of society."[36] While cancer is objectively an abnormal condition in that it threatens people's lives, the effects of its abnormality are also socially constructed, as cancer rhetorics aimed at saving lives exist alongside those that emphasize the need to ensure that the effects of the disease do not interfere with the proper functioning of society. The topoi of war, positivity, and prevention function at different historical moments to highlight personal health as operating within and to some extent subservient to a network of social concerns that include the preservation of a strong social and economic structure that contributes to the consistent progress of the whole.

This focus on progress illuminates the complex factors that define cancer's representation through public discourse and images that resonate broadly across the social spectrum. Leah Ceccarelli's study of the frontier metaphor in scientific discourse includes the insight that "metaphor can have a tremendous influence on what public policies we adopt and on our conceptions of ourselves and others, restricting our options to those that are conceivable within the imaginative constraints of the worldview being proferred by that specific language choice."[37] Part of this worldview invokes the values associated with masculinity, as Jackie Stacey notes in identifying the connections among cancer, power, and gender: "The desire for order and control, for permanence and immutability, produces a masculine drive to mark out the boundaries of a separate territory."[38] The impossibility of imagining social norms challenged by the unpredictability of cancer generates topoi that demonstrate how people can respond to the threat of cancer in ways that will ultimately maintain those norms despite what appears to be an irredeemable disruption of normality.

Intersections among the many faces of eugenics and illness are particularly pronounced in the emphasis on the vigor and productivity that are a necessary component of one's contribution to a thriving society. Brad Byrom's study of the rise of hospital-schools during the progressive era focuses on the way in which an emerging industrial economy shaped notions of disability during the early twentieth century: "The obligation of every male citizen was to work. Through work, men contributed to the economic well-being of the nation, set an example for younger generations, and symbolized the most prized aspect of the American character—independence."[39] In a similar vein, John Williams-Searle notes a connection between the ideal of productivity and masculinity, asking, "Why did working men conflate 'independence' (demonstrated by control over one's body, one's household, one's workplace, and one's financial well-being) with 'manliness'?"[40] K. Walter Hickel also notes the connection between economics and disability in his discussion of compensation for World War I veterans: "Federal lawmakers defined disability as functional impairment, a declension from a normal body or mind that reduced one's capacity for productive labor," which ultimately "revealed disability as an artifact of capitalist democracy, resonating throughout its economic, social, and political relations."[41]

The eugenic concern with disability as a drag on economic productivity extends to disabling conditions such as illness. Elof Axel Carlson notes that degeneracy theory, a linchpin of eugenic ideology, "found its origins in the urbanization surrounding the Industrial Revolution and the social problems created by the late nineteenth century's boom-bust economy. Accidents, ill health, and the tragedies of life . . . that could lead to unreliability at work or unemployment compounded the structural economic challenges that strained American life."[42] While Carlson's focus is on sterilization practices aimed at protecting society from the effects of inherited degeneracy, the less drastic effects of the concerns he outlines can be found in the cultural mandate to look past the bodies of those whose perceived weakness created "unreliability at work or unemployment,"[43] a threat to central components of the national ethos. This orientation includes in its purview not only people with disabilities but those whose chronic illnesses make it impossible to sustain the level of production that can be maintained by those who have the robust health manifested in the ideal citizen.

RHETORIC AND EUGENICS

Curing the diseases of people with illness is an altruistic aim, and the harsh eugenic practices perpetrated against the poor and disabled during the early twentieth century did not target people with chronic illnesses. Eugenic impulses are nevertheless evident in rhetoric that urges cancer patients to assert strength and positivity they may not possess. The primary audience for such arguments is not people with cancer but those who want to be assured that they can maintain an appropriate distance from a disease they fear. Similar strains can be seen in contemporary arguments pertaining to the COVID-19 pandemic. The death notices of COVID patients frequently include information about the health and preexisting medical conditions of those who have died, implicitly offering assurance that the threat is not as worrisome as we might fear since the disease most often affects those who are old and infirm and spares those who are young and strong. In various ways, a society influenced by eugenics conveys the message that any weakness that limits the contribution individuals can make to society ultimately undermines their worth, which further suggests that those who are productive contributors need not concern themselves with those who aren't. In this way, those who are healthy distance themselves from the threat of disability in order to "solidify their mutual membership in the realm of the normal."[44] The inflection of eugenics often subverts the educational purpose of public health rhetoric to establish a comforting distance between the sick and the well, ensuring that the disabling effects of illness do not unnecessarily disrupt "the realm of the normal."

This line of reasoning subtly pervades cancer rhetoric, even as many people involved in the move to publicize cancer would not have intended to make such problematic connections. Dominant cancer topoi do not feature arguments that people with cancer should be sterilized; they do, however, construct an idealized response to cancer aligned with the ascribed qualities valued by eugenics: powerful, resilient, productive, intelligent, and progressive. Such images often take hold and assume a life of their own. People who have been diagnosed with cancer are likely at some point to encounter at least one of many stock phrases that have become standard fare in discourses about cancer: "Just keep your spirits up—attitude is everything"; "You'll get through this—you're a fighter!"; "Were they able to catch it early?"; "Have you ever been a smoker?"; "You're so brave—I would just fall apart if I were in your place!"; "You're such an inspiration." Such statements come from people who mean well, often reflecting a desire to offer support in the face of an overwhelming sense of dread. And these comments are not entirely wrong: there is a place for vigilance, courage, and a hopeful outlook in the cancer experience. However, many people with cancer are keenly aware that such formulaic responses fall short of capturing the complexity of their experiences with the disease. They also implicitly provide an accepted range of responses that ostensibly support people with cancer but actually serve the purpose of reassuring an anxious public that cancer need not stand in the way of social progress, because the threat can be contained through determination and a healthy disposition.

Although the emergence of cancer rhetorics in the early twentieth century came about with the goal of promoting early detection through alleviating the shame and fear surrounding cancer, the intersections among these lines of argument and the cultural potency of eugenics creates a situation in which the visibility afforded by cancer rhetorics is filtered through a eugenic vision that subsumes the effects of cancer within powerful modern values that emphasize control and independence. A further dimension of this view includes the implicit assumption that vulnerability of any kind indicates flaws in the person with cancer. Carlson describes an early twentieth-century shift in eugenic thought relevant to understanding cancer topoi: "Instead of asking, 'Why does God allow bad things to happen to good people?' American intellectuals increasingly asked, 'What is it about an individual's inherent biology that makes him bad?'"[45] While people with cancer might be exempt from certain social stigmas levied against those who are disabled or are deemed racially, socially, or intellectually inferior, the complexity of their experiences has often been reduced to lines of argument that establish a normalized vision of individuals untouched by the most debilitating effects of the disease, which in turn implicitly assigns blame to those who experience the worst consequences of illness.

The argument that cancer rhetoric is infused with eugenic ideologies is grounded in the view that eugenics has constituted a fluid and evolving force in American society that extends beyond policies and actions into the formation of attitudes that subtly shape the language people use in describing conditions and experiences that deviate from narrow standards of normalcy. As Dolmage notes, "eugenics was a powerful rhetoric as well as a series of practices."[46] This book shows how the "powerful rhetoric" of eugenics, deployed across social and medical institutions that were in varying ways influenced by eugenic philosophies prominent during the period when the goal of publicizing cancer emerged, subtly influenced the development of cancer rhetorics, as the public was urged to respond to the potentially disabling effects of disease in ways that reflected the impulse to assert control over all disabling conditions. While it is certainly not my aim to question the admirable goal of eradicating cancer, it is important to note how easily the scientific zeal to pursue this worthy aim becomes subsumed within a dominant rhetorical framework focused on eliminating imperfection, promoting progress, maintaining control, and protecting civic fitness and productivity. As discourse about cancer moves from private to public life, from the home to institutions responsible for publicizing the disease, cancer is no longer exclusively a threat to the lives of individuals, but also becomes an enemy to the vitality of society as a whole. The emergence of dominant cancer topoi of war, positivity, and prevention may in varying degrees benefit people with cancer, but they are also inflected with a eugenic impulse that counters the threat of cancer not only through medical advances but also through the social control promised through the strong, healthy, and productive "people" constructed by cancer topoi. In this way, cancer topoi reflect genuine benefits of medical progress but also reflect the limits established by the existing "parameters of what 'the people' of that culture could possibly become."[47]

CANCER RHETORIC AND THE EUGENIC GAZE

The twentieth-century eugenic gaze replaces the shamed silence of the nineteenth century with rhetoric that makes cancer both visible and invisible, as cancer publicity suppresses the lived experiences of people with cancer in order to elevate eugenic claims of control and resilience. These recurring topoi and images generate a static and reassuring image of cancer that adheres to what Garland-Thomson describes as the process that takes place through the representation of the diverse identities and experiences of people with disabilities, which "frequently obscures these complexities in favor of the rhetorical or symbolical potential of the prototypical disabled figure, who often functions as a lightning rod for the pity, fear, discomfort, guilt, or sense of normalcy of the reader."[48] Although public cancer rhetoric functions differently from the literary representation of people with disabilities that is Garland-Thomson's focus, the two share common ground in containing the perceived threat associated with impairment by flattening the complexities of cancer in favor of images that can provide emotional release and reassurance. Cancer rhetoric therefore not only fulfills the ostensible objective of raising public awareness but also evokes emotional responses such as "horror, fear, pity, compassion, and avoidance" as a first step in managing what Lennard Davis describes as the "disruption" of disability that "must be regulated, rationalized, contained."[49]

Cancer constitutes sudden impairment that undermines the imagined invincibility that lies at the heart of the American ethos in a unique way. Garland-Thomson writes, "The category of disability exists as a way to exclude the kinds of bodily forms, functions, impairments, changes, or ambiguities that call into question our cultural fantasy of the body as a neutral, compliant, and predictable instrument of some transcendent will."[50] She further describes the tension between the strong interest in disability and the desire to maintain distance from it as grounded in its centrality as part of the human experience: "As a culture, we are at once obsessed with and intensely conflicted about the disabled body. We fear, deify, disavow, avoid, abstract, revere, conceal, and reconstruct disability—perhaps because it is one of the most universal, fundamental of human experiences. After all, we will all become disabled if we live long enough."[51] While Garland-Thomson is certainly accurate that "we will all become disabled if we live long enough," it is possible for people to take some comfort in the notion that the onset of disability might at least be delayed to the point where they have "lived long enough." In contrast, although cancer is most common among elderly people, it is generally known to affect people at every life stage and is frequently experienced as a sudden event that apparently comes out of nowhere. Statistics indicating how common cancer is, along with its capacity to affect people ranging from the very young to the very old, make cancer a particularly powerful threat to our "cultural fantasy." The intense impulse to "fear, deify, disavow, avoid, abstract, revere, conceal, and reconstruct" has strong relevance for cancer topoi, as well as disability rhetoric. Attention to the rhetorical construction of cancer therefore provides a path to a deeper understanding of what disease and disability mean in our society and how language reflects and structures our reality. In "Disability Rhetorics," Dolmage writes, "Disability rhetorics . . . are means of conceptualizing not just how meaning is attached to disability, but are means of conceptualizing the knowledge and meaning that disability *generates*."[52] To study the dissemination of particular lines of argument about cancer offers insight not only into patterns of argument that have defined its representation across decades but also into what these arguments reveal about cultural attitudes toward disease and impairment more broadly.

In pursuing an understanding of the complex evolution of cancer rhetoric across the twentieth century, I spent several years conducting research in archives from the Memorial Sloan Kettering Cancer Center Library and Archives (housed at the Rockefeller Archive Center), the Mary Lasker papers (housed at the Columbia University Rare Book and Manuscript Library), the National Library of Medicine, and the Historical Resources Center, Research Medical Library at the University of Texas MD Anderson Cancer Center. My study of a wide range of materials gathered there, including press releases, films, public service announcements, news clippings, radio and television scripts, correspondence, speeches, pamphlets and flyers, annual reports, and scrapbooks, along with additional secondary scholarship pertaining to cancer history, has enhanced my understanding of themes and patterns that have emerged in public cancer rhetoric at different historical moments. This rhetorical perspective yields insight about the frameworks that structure the possibilities for how cancer can be imagined. Mol writes, "To enact a disease is also to enact norms and standards. This is because the entity afflicted by the disease deviates—from some normality."[53] Cancer topoi have had a pervasive presence in modern life for so long that most people take these common lines of argument for granted. History helps to illuminate the complex workings of these topoi through situating them within the larger historical contexts from which they have emerged and interrogating the possibilities and limitations that the process of rhetorical classification and interpretation offer to the people who are created by cancer rhetorics.

My archival study of cancer rhetoric's twentieth-century development in the United States reveals the dynamic intersections among medicine, language, and public life across different historical moments and cultural contexts, offering what Segal describes as a "kairotic account of medical history."[54] Segal describes "kairology" as "a rhetorically tilted medical history," which generates insight not through uncovering new facts about medicine but instead through illuminating the integral role of persuasion in the development of that history.[55] A kairology of cancer rhetoric illuminates the role of language in both scientific developments and the public's understanding of the disease, supporting Lisa Keränen's interest in expanding the rhetoric of science to include "persuasion both in the conduct of science and in its circulation in public life."[56] The examination of cancer rhetoric as historically situated in changing environments and dynamic social relationships provides insight into how discourse shapes public and private perceptions of what it means to have cancer—and more broadly about the ways in which language shapes all human experience. A historical perspective reveals how cancer rhetorics emerge from specific cultural moments and are constructed by a complicated network of influences, illustrating Christa Teston's claim that "rhetoric is doing, or a way of performing the world materially."[57] The kairology that I have developed from these materials reveals cancer rhetoric as a forceful presence in developing public awareness about cancer and constructing a people who collectively establish an American disposition toward a ubiquitous and mysterious disease.

CANCER RHETORIC, CULTURAL ANXIETY, AND THE LIMITS OF INTERPRETATION

The historical study of the origins, resilience, and transformation of cancer topoi illuminates the intricate intersections among language, medicine, and culture. Because health is central to public life, the study of cancer rhetoric offers opportunities not only to understand cultural perspectives on cancer but also to examine the underlying anxieties that shape those perspectives. Siddhartha Mukherjee writes, "Every era casts illness in its own image. Society, like the ultimately psychosomatic patient, matches its medical afflictions to its psychological crises; when a disease touches such a visceral chord, it is often because that chord is already resonating."[58] To understand the cultural relationship between society and disease is to understand much about how rhetoric functions in different cultural moments. As Dolmage notes, "Studying any culture's attitudes and arguments about the body always connects us intimately with attitudes and arguments about rhetorical possibility. That is, to care about the body is to care about how we make meaning."[59] Cancer has historically served as a particularly visible emblem of that which people fear and desire to contain, evident in a 1913 address by Curtis E. Lakeman, executive director of the American Society for the Control of Cancer, in which cancer is described as "the mystery of medicine, the veritable sphinx of disease."[60] This book's consideration of the unfolding of the rhetorical possibilities that are deployed in order to make meaning of the disease, to solve a mystery that appears to be unsolvable, will consistently engage with the question of what cultural values influence and constrain those possibilities, as well as how particular rhetorical choices shape public understanding and experiences with the disease.

My hope is that a kairology of cancer rhetoric can illuminate the ways in which the active pursuit of a normate society significantly influenced by eugenic ideologies has not only affected the lives of cancer patients but also shaped the public's view of what disease and disability mean. The persistent deployment of themes of control and containment in cancer rhetoric reflects and contributes to broader cultural perspectives that are also relevant to people with disabilities, people who have illnesses other than cancer, and people who are neither ill nor disabled. As Davis notes, "Just as the conceptualization of race, class, and gender shapes the lives of those who are not black, poor, or female, so the concept of disability regulates the bodies of those who are 'normal.'"[61] Davis insists that this recognition requires that we "understand and theorize the discourse of disability, to see that the object of disability studies is not the person using the wheelchair or the Deaf person but the set of social, historical, economic, and cultural processes that regulate and control the way we think about and think through the body."[62] Davis's call resonates with Dolmage's insistence "that the experience of disability . . . allows for a more real (inherently unstable) perspective on embodiment and, through embodiment, a more real perspective on rhetoric and our cunning world."[63] An examination of the particular ways in which eugenic ideologies shape cancer discourses can illuminate patterns of normalizing bodies that take place in other contexts, as well. It can also make us aware of the complex impulses that drive us to isolate and remove from public view those who are most vulnerable during periods of heightened awareness about the uncertainty that is a constant feature of all matters pertaining to human health. US cancer publicity emerged during a period defined both by this awareness and by a determined resolve to believe in the power of science, in partnership with business and industry, to overcome even the most significant challenges to the health and prosperity of the nation. The tension between the goal of awareness and the persistent assertion of national strength lies at the heart of cancer rhetoric, as well as many other examples of US public health rhetoric.

Subsequent chapters will explore in detail the dynamic interactions among cancer rhetoric and the broad range of participants who contribute to and are influenced by it. This investigation will focus on key topoi that respond to a disease that is persistently at the forefront of the public's consciousness—and that in turn not only constitute the identities of cancer patients and the medical community but also establish a people prepared to combat the disease through awareness, strength of will, and resilience. Chapter 1 traces the emergence of cancer publicity in the early decades of the twentieth century and explores how this goal intersects with the flourishing of eugenic organizations and ideologies in the scientific community as well as more broadly in US cultural life. The 1913 formation of the American Society for the Control of Cancer (ASCC), which later became the American Cancer Society, can be seen as a catalyst for the view that early detection and successful treatment of cancer depend upon publicity. This emphasis creates a dynamic tension, as the long-standing impulse to maintain secrecy about the disease is challenged by medical and social developments that emphasize the need to publicize cancer in order to educate the public and pursue research funding. This historical perspective illuminates the benefits and risks that come from breaking the silence about cancer, as publicity makes possible the desired goals of public awareness and increased financial support but also sets the stage for representations of cancer that at times subsume, regulate, and, to a certain extent, commodify the experiences and identities of cancer patients. In this way, silence, publicity, and eugenic impulses converge, as efforts to make cancer visible are consistently shaped by cultural values that ensure that circulating representations of cancer emphasize progress and self-sufficiency guided by science and industrial development.

This tension in the goals and outcomes of cancer publicity are reflected in the emergence of topoi that offer possible responses to the fearful specter of the disease. Chapter 2 discusses the complex factors that shape the emphasis on war as a metaphor relevant to government policy, medical research, and personal experience. As referenced earlier, the ASCC was formed in 1913, the beginning of a period in which war was on the minds of most Americans. Many early cancer researchers had ties to the military, and a number of advances in cancer treatment came about through their experiences there. While the information disseminated by the ASCC was firmly grounded in facts available to the medical professionals who were its founders, the strategy of metaphorically linking cancer and war was the result of several complementary impulses. First, it reflected the material links between medical research and the military. It also connected with the public's preoccupation with war, a concern that continued to be prominent across decades defined by two world wars. In addition, war metaphors captured the eugenic desire to conquer those components of human experience that were seen as a danger to the goal of progress. While this metaphor offers the potential of empowering patients in what they may in fact experience as a battle, its connection with broader cultural conceptions of disease as failure reflects the eugenic ideologies that were dominant during this period.

Even as cancer patients are consistently depicted as fierce warriors, the early medical view that black bile causes both cancer and melancholy also has a significant presence in twentieth-century cancer topoi. The third chapter traces the evolution of cancer's perceived connection with melancholy in modern topoi that urge cancer patients to seize control of their disease through a positive outlook. This historical perspective identifies positive dimensions of this line of argument's challenge to earlier depictions of the negative and hopeless plight of cancer patients, but it also points toward problematic assumptions that evolve from connecting cancer recovery with a patient's personal disposition and desire for health. The persistent suggestion that those who have the personal and material resources to develop a disposition impervious to the damage of cancer has strong eugenic overtones, reinforcing a social vision of a world in which only those who are deemed deficient, in this case in their inability to maintain the right kind of outlook, will be troubled by the worst effects of disease.

By midcentury, the turn toward research that identified potential causes of cancer called for a new emphasis on prevention, which was taken up in various ways by the medical community, cancer advocacy groups, and the public at large. While this area of focus led to material benefits, the topos of prevention, like lines of argument linking cancer to positivity, has important implications that go beyond the facts of medical research. Chapter 4 explores how the goal of prevention generated new ways of talking about cancer that have problematic implications alongside the potential benefits associated with public awareness. On one hand, new information about cancer risk factors saved lives by usefully illuminating the links between cancer and particular behaviors and environmental conditions. On the other hand, the emphasis on prevention rhetorically constructs "the people" affected by public health as having uniform access to medical knowledge and the socioeconomic resources to minimize risk. These discourses bring into sharp relief the raced, classed, and gendered fault lines that have functioned in cancer discourses since the twentieth century, as well as the ways in which a eugenic orientation suggests that cancer diagnosis is a matter of personal responsibility. This shift threatens to reinscribe earlier images of cancer as shameful, as discourses of prevention might be interpreted as suggesting that adequate vigilance, personal intelligence, or a significantly disciplined health regimen might nearly eliminate the danger of cancer—a view that implicitly suggests that those who develop cancer might in some way hold responsibility for their plight.

But the public dissemination of information about cancer through organizations, institutions, and the media is not only the only story about cancer to be told. The fifth and concluding chapter gestures to the fact that people with cancer have their own stories to tell, a phenomenon that has achieved greater prominence through the rise of social media in the decades subsequent to this book's focus. While people with cancer often draw from cancer topoi in documenting their own experiences, the substantial proliferation and expansion of writings in recent years highlight the diverse identities and experiences encompassed within the realm of cancer and complicate what was in an earlier era a more totalizing eugenic depiction of cancer's character and effects. While they are of course not totally detached from the cultural constraints within which they're situated, the perspectives of cancer patients foster attention to the multiplicity of what it means to live with cancer and to the material reality of experiences that cannot be easily assimilated into a eugenic vision of masculine health, prosperity, and productivity. The willingness to see cancer as a complex human experience offers a pathway for cancer rhetorics grounded in mutuality, support, and care.

1

Publicizing Cancer

EUGENIC VISIBILITY

Understanding the tension between the impulses to make cancer visible and to suppress the complex reality of what cancer entails begins with situating the emergence of cancer rhetoric within a larger cultural context. As discussed in the introduction, cancer rhetoric persuasively created a people informed and equipped to respond to the disease in a way that would preserve modern social progress, a central value in the early twentieth-century United States. As is generally the case, the rhetorical construction of the people bounds "what 'the people' of that culture could possibly become."[1] By the same token, this process inevitably entails working within and subtly adapting to established cultural constraints in order to transform and prepare people to face the challenges of the situation. While cancer had existed for centuries, a society grounded in science and modernity demanded a new response, one that would bring cancer into public view without disrupting confidence in the people's capacity to pursue a more nearly perfect society.

Many areas of US public life in the early decades of the twentieth century were defined by the determination to *know*—and the belief that knowledge would inevitably point toward solutions to social problems that stood in the way of progress. During this period, the highly prized pursuit of knowledge was supported through scientific breakthroughs in many areas, including disease and genetics. But acquiring knowledge was not enough; the public needed to be apprised of the latest information in order to participate in the collective pursuit of a better society. The goal of making knowledge available accounts for the shift from the silence about cancer typical of the nineteenth century to the more aggressive pursuit of publicity as a central feature of cancer rhetoric from the early twentieth century forward. In describing the impetus for the establishment of the ASCC in 1913, historian Walter Ross notes that prior to that time, the disease "was not named in polite society" due to the fact that cancer "ranked in shame with syphilis and other unmentionable afflictions."[2] The perceived benefit of making visible those fears that had previously been kept in the shadows is one of many instances of the aggressive pursuit of information that was a characteristic feature of the early twentieth century.

A seemingly natural accompaniment to the pursuit of knowledge was a heightened interest in classification, which was seen as a good in itself but was particularly useful in facilitating intervention in those circumstances that departed from the norm. This outlook had particular consequences for people with disabling conditions that differed from those of previous generations. Henri-Jacques Stiker contrasts the heightened focus on disability in the modern era with the Middle Ages, when disability was a private matter that was assumed to be part of human experience: "The chronically ill were spontaneously part of the world and of a society that was accepted as being multifaceted, diversified, disparate. The kind of social eugenics that was to be the fate of recent society had not yet emerged. . . . This was more than tolerance; it was real life, with which one compromised as best one could, without wishing to change it by various techniques and various treatments, and without wishing to exclude it either."[3]

Thus, the process of making difference visible, while ostensibly helpful in raising awareness of disease and disability, had the unintended effect of supporting the emergence of eugenic ideologies dedicated to eliminating those differences that threatened the goal of progress. The ideal of social progress, supported by the heightened capacity for diagnosis, classification, and treatment, moved the focus from the acceptance of life's ills toward action to mitigate or prevent them. Stiker's insight can be extended from the focus on disability to include disease and impairment. Removing cancer from the shadows and promoting heightened awareness undoubtedly saved lives, but it also entailed participation in a system of classification that had less positive consequences, as the goal of making illness visible signaled the removal of affected individuals from the bustling "normality" of modern life.

Stiker's depiction of the modern focus on classifying and isolating difference includes the notion that this process expands the number of disabling conditions, "because the basic social fabric will less and less preserve the affected individual and will label more and more people."[4] His assessment that the expansion of disability is accompanied by the shrinking of the acceptable norm is also relevant to the evolution of cancer rhetoric, which follows a similar pattern in illuminating the ubiquitous presence of cancer while inadvertently widening the gap between sickness and health and reinscribing the desirability of a narrowly defined norm: "Every failure to adjust will be labeled a disability. We are caught in a process that is almost insane: the least maladjustment will be catalogued, referenced, and made into a disability, which will in turn entail specific measures, even initiate some very specialized programs before deficient adjustment is declared normalizable. If we take into account elderly persons especially, we could almost say that the vast majority of the population will be disabled, with the social norm taking refuge in a small number of individuals. This normal individual will preferentially be white, male, young, healthy, handsome, educated, and . . . submissive!"[5] Because cancer is often a temporarily disabling condition, cancer topoi serve the purpose of classifying the obvious abnormality of cancer and providing a verbal mechanism for overcoming its effects as soon as possible, part of a process by which "deficient adjustment is declared normalizable."[6] Cancer rhetoric therefore supplements medical treatment aimed at restoring physical health, offering a framework for suppressing the abnormality that is an almost certain result of a cancer diagnosis.

This process begins with images that provide a hypervisible outlet for confronting social anxiety and then are managed, through the use of cancer topoi, in ways that reinforce the claim that, even under the worst possible conditions, normality, defined in terms of a vigorous, white, healthy, and active lifestyle, can prevail. The economic underpinnings of normality are evident early in the century and continue to be a feature of contemporary life, as A. Suresh Canagarajah notes: "The search for perfection reaches an exaggerated scale in our current neoliberal political dispensation. The market functions on the assumption that individuals have unlimited capacity for self-improvement or even self-invention. People are expected to constantly reinvent themselves in relation to the knowledge and skills valued by the market."[7]

The lines of argument that describe how people with cancer should reinvent themselves illuminate specific ways in which a eugenic gaze normalizes the abnormality of cancer by elevating the qualities of courage, cheerful positivity, and the proactive pursuit of better health—the kinds of qualities that might be possessed by the modern individual that Stiker describes as the imaginary cultural norm.[8] The irony underlying the early twentieth-century goal of eliminating the shame of cancer is that the impulse to control and normalize people's experiences with the disease ultimately generated a new form of the shame, silence, and invisibility that had been dominant features of cancer rhetoric in the nineteenth century. All of these lines of argument raise questions about the genetic deficiencies and personal qualities that might explain cancer's origins, as well as the insidious suggestion that people have the potential to overcome the horrifying effects of cancer through the right attitude and conduct.

EUGENICS AND TWENTIETH-CENTURY AMERICAN THOUGHT

As discussed in the introduction, the emergence of cancer rhetoric in the early decades of the twentieth century corresponds with the period in which eugenics became a prominent part of US cultural and intellectual life. Both cancer rhetoric and eugenic ideologies are based in the pursuit of a public commitment to improve the lives of individuals and the health of society. Both also share an emphasis on the capacity of scientific knowledge to promote the goals of public health and social progress. But both have a dark side accompanying these ostensibly positive goals. The obvious evil of eugenics lies in the argument that it is permissible to pursue progress at any cost, which includes practices aimed at eliminating the genetic lines perceived as interfering with the broader goals of health and social improvement. While the damaging consequences of popular cancer topoi are less obvious, there is embedded in the emphasis on power, knowledge, and progress an impulse to suppress those identities and experiences that undermine dominant representations of medical and personal achievements in managing the disease.

In pointing out these historic connections, I am by no means arguing that everyone involved in cancer research and advocacy was also involved in eugenics. Certainly, there are significant ways in which eugenics had nothing to do with cancer research or the project of making cancer more publicly visible. However, it is also impossible to ignore ways in which eugenic concerns permeate arguments about cancer, in part due to the convergence between eugenics and early genetic research as well as to the eugenic vision of social progress that was so much a part of public life during the period in which cancer publicity came into being. This insight is particularly significant in light of the fact that the public's acceptance of eugenic ideologies is based in part on the appropriation of science to promote troubling cultural assumptions about genetics, racial purity, and intellectual progress. The power of these assumptions can be found through their circulation across social institutions outside of the laboratories and hospitals that implemented eugenic procedures such as genetic classification and sterilization. As I argued in the introduction, although these eugenic practices are not directly relevant to cancer rhetoric, the prominence and ubiquity of eugenics in the early twentieth-century United States and the imbrication of eugenics, science, and corporate life calls for careful consideration in analyzing cancer rhetoric, particularly as it helps to account for the continuing strains of anxiety that shape those discourses that ostensibly came into being to replace shame and silence with visibility and hope.

MAKING CANCER VISIBLE: THE AMERICAN SOCIETY FOR THE CONTROL OF CANCER

Many of the early arguments for publicizing cancer were grounded in the assumption that people could be empowered through knowledge. In his preface to the 1907 publication *The Control of a Scourge, Or How Cancer Is Curable*, British surgeon C. P. Childe describes his book as "an attempt, however imperfect, to substitute for ignorance and despair, sound knowledge and hope."[9] Childe acknowledges that public discussion of cancer "offends our sense of delicacy" and might also heighten fear but insists that the benefits of an educated public outweigh the risks.[10] Childe's determination to make information about cancer accessible signals the emerging conviction that a reasoned presentation of factual information to the public has a major role in the medical community's success in treating cancer.[11]

The effort to create a concerted public response to cancer was substantially facilitated by the formation of the American Society for the Control of Cancer. ASCC executive director Curtis E. Lakeman signaled this organization's emphasis on publicity in a 1913 address to the National Conference of Charities and Correction, where he informed his audience of his intention "to ask you to consider the problem of cancer not from the medical point of view, but in its aspect of increasing importance as a social question calling for definite social intervention."[12] According to Lakeman, the society's statement of purpose in shaping the "social intervention" included maintaining data about cancer, developing networks of communication among those engaged in its study and treatment, and sharing information to promote early detection and treatment.

The ASCC's rhetorical tactics, influenced by its ties to the medical and corporate communities, initially utilized facts and statistics as the basis to motivate action. The ASCC's statistics committee chair, Frederick L. Hoffman of the Prudential Insurance Company, became an important voice in the organization's early development. The emphasis on acquiring statistics about cancer reflected the ASCC's stated purpose, which again emphasized the intrinsic value available through information: "To disseminate knowledge concerning the symptoms, diagnosis, treatment and prevention of cancer, to investigate the conditions under which cancer is found and to compile statistics in regard thereto."[13] Although Hoffman was not himself a scientist involved in cancer research, he asserted the importance of data in the cause of cancer prevention and treatment. In this way, the early communication of the ASCC illustrates Carolyn Miller's argument that scientific rhetoric relies on "technical ethos," which establishes authority through a self-effacing reliance on facts, as "the favoring of logos becomes its own ethos."[14] This pattern is evident in Hoffman's white paper titled "The Statistical Evidence of the Increase in Cancer," which argues that statistics are as valuable in cancer research as work done in the laboratory: "It would also seem far better to give encouragement to every form of statistical research into the cancer problem particularly as regards the ascertained value of different methods of medical and surgical treatment, than to give over emphasis to the experimental method or laboratory research, which, even though it succeeded in the discovery of the causes or the cures of cancer would still, as in the case of tuberculosis, fail for many years to affect a very considerable reduction in the death rate."[15] While statistical information about cancer furthered public awareness of the disease, the emphasis on objectivity and generalizable conclusions established a framework for visibility that inevitably obscured the particularities that shape individuals' experiences with disease. It also established a pattern in which methods for assessing and communicating about cancer carried a rhetorical weight that paralleled the more tangible benefits available from laboratory research and developments in treatment.

In addition to his altruistic aims, Hoffman's position with Prudential led him to consider how cancer statistics might be used to design appeals attentive to corporate goals, and he used this strategy in arguing that improvements in detection and treatment would hold immediate financial benefits. In a 1913 letter to insurance company presidents, Hoffman wrote, "It requires no argument to convince you that a reduction in the cancer death rate must, of necessity, affect most favorably the mortality experience of your Company, with resulting pecuniary benefits to your policyholder, to say nothing of the incalculable value of such a campaign from a humanitarian point of view."[16] The effort to make cancer publicly visible was from the beginning focused on the immediate goal of health, but the message was shaped by varied appeals to dominant American values, which assumed seamless connections among sound reasoning, corporate solvency, public health, and social prosperity and progress.

At the same time, the need to situate logic within a larger argument that would appeal to the public was clear to those who were involved in making the case for greater public attention to the disease. The effort to disseminate medical and scientific information effectively was complicated. Historian James T. Patterson notes that the ASCC faced an ongoing dilemma in its publicity efforts: "If they put out sober messages about the virtues of early detection and medical intervention, they ran the risk of boring their audience. But if they tried to dramatize things by emphasizing the horrors of the disease. . . they might be accused of frightening people."[17] Across ensuing years of the organization's development, the ASCC worked to balance education and fear. Even the apparently uncontroversial distribution of printed materials containing four warning signs of cancer, launched in 1919, was considered problematic by those who maintained earlier assumptions that cancer was not a suitable subject for public discussion.[18] In 1921 the *Journal of the American Medical Association* characterized the warning signs as likely "to arouse in a certain number of persons phobias almost as terrifying as the disease feared."[19] S. Lochlann Jain argues that the effort to spark public awareness of the threat of cancer without creating alarm generated persistent lines of argument that offered reassurance that implicitly created new pressures: "Early-detection narratives, suggesting future and past counterfactuals, seek to break the deeply held association between cancer and death with one simple directive: *You won't die if you just see your doctor!* The directive has a foreboding undertone: *It could have been different.* We can change the course of history—and if we can't now because we waited too long, we could have before."[20]

ASCC leaders appear to have been keenly aware of the challenges surrounding their project as they pursued their resolve to bring cancer into public view. Their determination to manage this challenge was based in the conviction that publicizing cancer held material benefits that would save lives. The optimism surrounding this goal is evident in a 1943 ASCC publication titled "Cancer and Public Relations," which places public awareness on a par with medical developments in cancer research: "One of the heartening phases of the war on cancer is the development of public relations work. Reinforcing surgery, radium, and the x-ray, publicity is a powerful weapon in the arsenal reared against the disease."[21] Many cancer advocates also understood that one step in improving the plight of cancer patients was to overcome the fear that had historically interfered with progress, a point that was succinctly illustrated in the 1946 *New York Herald Tribune* headline: "We Can't Cure Cancer by Shuddering!"[22]

In addition to its own outlets, the ASCC used the information it acquired to support the dissemination of information about cancer by the media. Kirsten E. Gardner notes that the organization produced several of its own publications within the first year of its founding but also actively encouraged magazines to publish articles about cancer. She describes the development of publications such as *Hygeia,* which the AMA began in 1923 with the goal of communicating medical developments to the general public, as part of "an increasingly evident twentieth-century trend—the blurring of boundaries between medical and popular literature and between a professional and lay audience."[23] Although the "sane, scientific articles" published in *Hygeia* reflected the ASCC's central educational goals, the organization also recognized that the effort to spark public attention sometimes required more than strictly logical appeals.[24]

In addition to engaging with audiences through logic and emotion, arguments about cancer also illustrate rhetoric's persistent tendency to appeal to dominant cultural values. During the same period when the ASCC was charting its course, eugenic ideologies were taking strong hold among scientists and the American public, and those interested in expanding the public's appreciation for eugenics faced similar issues in determining how to package what they considered to be important scientific information to an uninformed public. While the most visible evil of eugenics is evident in the use of science to limit the growth of a population deemed undesirable, the prominence of eugenic thought and its support from the scientific community was sustained in more insidious forms through widespread belief in what at face value appeared to be more benign goals, including social measures aimed at creating a more healthy society, a goal that was based on an unstated vision of social progress bounded by particular assumptions about race and class. A key principle of the initiative, sometimes referred to as positive eugenics, focused on what Diane B. Paul and James Moore describe as the capacity of families "to enhance their biological fortunes through education, exercise, good nourishment, and the pursuit of 'higher' pleasures such as music and art."[25] The commitment of individuals and families to do their part in the formation of a better society provided an important foundation for practices that would also promote such enhancements, a project that would ultimately generate visible signs of social progress.[26]

While doing one's part to combat cancer is in some respects distinct from the cultural enrichment programs Paul and Moore describe, there are parallels to be found in assumptions about health, individual responsibility, and social progress that underlie cancer rhetoric. The dominance of these ideas is not surprising in light of the fact that during the early decades of the twentieth century, the American public was thoroughly immersed in discourses that established intricate connections among science, health and fitness, eugenics, and the well-being of society. In *World of Fairs: The Century-of-Progress Exhibitions,* Robert W. Rydell makes note of the complex ways in which world's fairs, an institution that had remarkable prominence in shaping American thought during the early decades of the twentieth century, collectively reinscribed these ideological links: "Woven into the dream world of goods was a hierarchical continuum of material and racial progress that signified nothing so much as the distance traveled from 'savagery' to 'civilization.' And, in a world alive with social-Darwinian ideas of evolution, displays of material and natural abundance became an outward sign of inward racial 'fitness' and culture."[27] For this reason, Rydell argues that world's fair exhibitions constituted an ideal medium for disseminating eugenic ideas.[28]

Science played an important role in persuading the public to appreciate the value of eugenic philosophy, a connection evident in the focus of the prominent science exhibits at world's fairs. According to Rydell, these exhibits "were intended to exemplify 'the idea of scientific and industrial unity' and to inject 'system' and 'order' into the exposition and, by extension, into American culture as a whole."[29] Rydell demonstrates various ways in which the pursuit of progress established an alliance among world's fair organizing committees, science, corporations, and eugenicists: "At both the Chicago and New York fairs, scientists sought to accomplish much more than the simple transmission of scientific information. . . . Many scientists who participated in the fairs pursued another goal as well, namely, to teach Americans that scientific and technological progress toward a future perfect world required large corporations and that judgements about what constituted progress could be left to the scientists themselves or to their corporate sponsors. Although they left Americans ill-prepared to confront the complexities of the dawning nuclear age, scientists involved in the fairs did construct the intellectual scaffolding—the normative discourse—that served to perpetuate the corporation-run state into the postwar period."[30] The normative discourse of science and corporate America provided a strong pathway for Americans to adopt eugenic frameworks that had the appearance of a forward-thinking mindset based in the ideals of progress and prosperity. Striking parallels exist between these frameworks for constructing alliances among scientific research, corporate enterprise, and a progressive society and arguments about the unique American capacity to overcome the threat of cancer.

In addition to the troubled connection between cancer rhetoric and eugenics, the emerging awareness of cancer's link to genetics created a symbiotic relationship between eugenics and cancer research, a connection that is subtly reflected in the language people used to describe the goal of overcoming the problem of cancer. These connections were supported through a degree of overlap between the community of scientific researchers and proponents of eugenics. In tracing the dissemination of eugenic thought and scientific innovation through the mechanism of world's fairs, Rydell highlights the work of individuals who were positioned to demonstrate the linkages across ideologies through the roles they inhabited. The 1915 Panama-Pacific International Exposition set aside a week for the theme of "race betterment" that included a conference organized by the Race Betterment Foundation, whose officers included Harvard University president emeritus Charles W. Eliot and Charles B. Davenport, director of the Cold Spring Harbor Laboratory.[31] Davenport's ambitions spurred him to take the lead in urging the Permanent International Eugenics Committee to hold the Second International Congress of Eugenics in New York City in 1921, and he went on to found the International Federation of Eugenics Organizations in 1925.[32]

One of the Cold Spring Harbor staff members Davenport recruited to assist with preparations for the event was director of research and noted cancer researcher C. C. Little, who worked at Cold Spring Harbor from 1919 until his appointment as president of the University of Maine in 1922. After moving from Maine to become president of the University of Michigan in 1925, Little returned to his focus on cancer research in 1929, when he founded the Jackson Laboratory in Bar Harbor. That same year, he agreed to become part-time managing director of the ASCC, a position he held until 1945. Little's instrumental role in a number of cancer initiatives included service as president of the American Association for Cancer Research in 1931 and 1940, collaboration with the Federation of Women's Clubs to establish the ASCC's Women's Field Army against Cancer, and assistance with writing and defending the National Cancer Institute Act. His commitment to eugenics recently led to the removal of his name from buildings at the University of Maine and the University of Michigan, along with an auditorium at the Jackson Lab, which he founded in 1929.[33]

Like other cancer advocates of his day, Little envisioned his role as providing the public with abundant information about cancer in ways that directly countered the silence of the past. In "Cancer Can Be Cured," Little uses the dark past as a backdrop for a more hopeful message about education's potential to facilitate a more enlightened understanding of cancer: "Once cancer was a word spoken only in whispers. It was taboo. People ranked it with tuberculosis in the days when that was called the 'white plague.' They were ashamed if it struck their family, hesitant to call a physician. They kept news of their affliction to themselves, going to a doctor only when driven by desperation."[34] He explicitly connects this shame with the ignorance and sense of hopelessness that limited cancer treatment in the past: "Most of the time, they did not recognize the symptoms. Often, if they did recognize them, they were so sure it was incurable, that they kept their secret to themselves, morbidly convinced that their death warrant had been signed."[35] While Little suggests that public discourse about cancer creates a much brighter picture in terms of survival rates, he also cautions that there is continued need for vigilance and education: "Although the taboo has been broken and cancer is openly talked about, written about and even filmed, there are still vast numbers of people who don't know, and may lose their lives because they don't know, these simple truths."[36] Little's notion of "simple truths" reinforces the argument that individuals hold their fate in their hands and that the danger cancer poses to "vast numbers" is largely due to their ignorance of the importance of early detection. The article ends with a list of facts about cancer, including possible symptoms, the benefits of early detection, and assurance that the disease is not contagious—a catalogue of material presented as a source of empowerment for patients.

Of course, Little was correct in his belief that information about cancer could play a positive role in saving lives by encouraging people to pursue necessary medical intervention. However, the progressive themes in Little's research in genetics and cancer and his interest in the ASCC's mission of educating the public about cancer prevention function alongside the problematic strains of eugenic thought that are another part of his legacy. As secretary-general of the Second International Congress of Eugenics, Little worked with other Cold Spring Harbor colleagues to advance the cause of both science and eugenics through what Rydell describes as an event that "confirmed eugenicists in their zeal to transmit the gospel of eugenics to a wider mass audience."[37] This cause was furthered through the recruitment of able volunteers such as Dr. Florence Brown Sherbon and Mary T. Watts, who collaborated on the development of competitions at state fairs that judged babies and families based on qualities deemed scientifically preferable in the preservation of a strong society.[38] In a letter to Davenport circa 1924, Watts wrote, "All I dare to hope for from our crude plan is the opening of a way for scientific facts to filter into the consciousness of the masses and then the people will save themselves."[39]

The eugenic goal of empowering people to "save themselves" through science hauntingly resonates with cancer rhetorics of the same period. After assuring the audience at the 1915 Public Meeting on the Control of Cancer that cancer is not contagious and may not be hereditary, Curtis E. Lakeman adds, "It is purely a question of the individual and his strength of mind and will to take care of himself."[40] An address by Edward Reynolds to the Massachusetts State Federation of Women's Clubs tellingly titled "Cancer a Controllable Disease: How the Women's Clubs Can Help the Less Intelligent" begins, "You ladies represent an enormous number of women who have been in effect automatically selected from the community as the possessors of intelligence and public spirit."[41] Although the eugenic goal of creating a people empowered to save themselves through science has important differences from the desire of medical researchers and advocates to promote public health through knowledge about the threat of cancer, the rhetorical construction of a people poised to address the debilitating effects of cancer through "strength of mind and will" and "intelligence and public spirit" strikingly resonates with the eugenic vision of social progress in the hands of the strong and intelligent.

The links between eugenics and cancer topoi are most evident in the widespread cultural anxiety surrounding any weakness that might undermine the eugenic vision of strength and progress. Advances in genetics, which were an important feature of cancer research, were motivated by the desire to ferret out those tendencies that potentially lead to abnormalities, including both disability and disease. Elof Axel Carlson notes that developments in medical research during the 1920s included "uncertainty among the leading lights in medical health and genetics about the relationship among 'degeneracy,' 'feeblemindedness,' disease susceptibility, and genetics."[42] Rudolf Virchow, the nineteenth-century German pathologist who was the first to identify cancer's origin in defective cells, made a number of valuable contributions to public health through his determination to connect medicine and politics. At the same time, Carlson describes Virchow's public hygiene movement, which became a cornerstone of German medical education, as a point of interest for physicians in the United States whose study with Virchow and his students provided a foundation for exploring how the notion of genetic disease prevention might be applied to the elimination of deficiencies through measures such as forced sterilization.[43]

While genetic researchers in the late nineteenth and early twentieth centuries investigated measures that might prevent the development of disease and other medical deficiencies, the public also had a role in adopting a lifestyle that would protect them from the worst effects of disease. In her study of self-improvement literature of the 1930s, Susan Currell argues that the growing interest in measures to cultivate personal strength emerged in response to the Great Depression, which was seen as a symbol of a society out of control, defined by "a national weakness and debility" and in need of strong leadership.[44] An important vehicle for disseminating this ideology was *Physical Culture* magazine, which Currell describes as a publication whose foundation in "will-power and science" became particularly popular during the Great Depression, "when illness and decay appeared to have infected the social fabric of the nation itself."[45] The magazine advocated "euthenics," an emphasis on health measures that could not only strengthen individuals but also promote gradual improvement in the "American racial stock."[46] Currell notes that euthenic goals of conquering disease and reversing social decline were captured in an April 1932 article highlighting Franklin Delano Roosevelt's "determined conquest" of polio and in the motto of founder Bernarr Macfadden: "Sickness is a sin; don't be a sinner. Weakness is a crime; don't be a criminal."[47] While Currell acknowledges that the exercise program advocated by Macfadden and supported by FDR appears to be grounded in a vision of modernity unrelated to the selective breeding program that is the most visible feature of eugenics, she argues that "the rhetoric of recovery and planning at that time shows that the self-improvement formula actually engaged closely with the eugenic thought of the 1930s."[48] According to Currell, the goals of the "euthenics" orientation of *Physical Culture* entailed "increasing human efficiency and health by improving the way humans interacted with and controlled their environment."[49] Currell makes a persuasive case for the complementary relationship between the euthenics promotion of health and fitness and eugenic measures, both of which were seamlessly woven into the fabric of society, as she notes that "eugenic ideas appeared to be in step with modern times and the national adjustment to a welfare state. Anti-eugenicists thus appeared old-fashioned, backward, and out of step with modern medical thinking."[50] The links between euthenics and the eugenic emphasis on social progress are not necessarily guiding forces in all of cancer research during this period, but the arguments for control and a progressive response to the problem of cancer enacted through cancer topoi often reflect the euthenic approach that Currell describes.

The goal of euthenics may have been to offer the reassurance that health is within the control of individuals committed to overcoming any health challenges they might encounter, but Currell notes that the outcome was more complicated: "It was ironic, therefore, that the quest for a healthier and more modern population also triggered intensified fears of further eugenic decay."[51] Cancer rhetoric reveals an intricate relationship between expressions of intense fear and the insistence that health challenges can be readily addressed through strength of will and proper health measures, demonstrating the conflicting cultural impulses Garland-Thomson describes as a simultaneous obsession with and desire for distance from disability.[52]

Part of the anxiety stemming from cancer related to the fact that it defied the eugenic vision that had comfortably located disease in populations who were vulnerable due to lack of proper hygiene and medical care. The extensive use of statistics in early cancer rhetoric reflected an appreciation for this scientific method of documenting modern social trends, but the statistical information about cancer troubled the paradigm of civilization as the sure path to health and progress. A 1913 address delivered to the National Conference of Charities and Correction by Curtis E. Lakeman, executive director of the ASCC, contains an extensive representation of measurable factors that point toward environmental causes affecting particular populations. Lakeman notes, "Cancer is rare among primitive races and most common among civilized people living under better material conditions. It appears to be more common among the well to do than the poor, and less common among persons below the average weight. During the period of slavery cancer was rare among negroes in the United States but since emancipation the cancer death rate has increased rapidly until now some forms of the disease at certain ages are more common among negroes than among whites."[53] Lakeman concludes that various factors, including "continued irritation," along with changes in environment and nutrition, may contribute to the development of cancer.

Of course, Lakeman's analysis does not consider obvious factors that might explain the rise in cancer among Black people after slavery, such as an increased life span and access to medical testing. However, the statistical evidence suggesting that cancer thrives in civilization helps explain one reason for the public anxiety surrounding the disease. Not only was cancer fearsome because of its frequency and lethal nature, but the statistical evidence proving that cancer was also "most common among civilized people" threatened the reassuring line of reasoning that governed typical eugenic discourses of that era. As referenced in the introduction, the construction of disability creates distance from "the kinds of bodily forms, functions, impairments, changes, or ambiguities that call into question our cultural fantasy of the body as a neutral, compliant, and predictable instrument of some transcendent will."[54] Eugenics helped establish that distance by assuring those who aligned themselves with the physical and mental ideal that they were participating in society's progress toward realizing the "cultural fantasy of the body," in contrast with members of the population who were deficient. Publicly focused cancer rhetoric came into being in an era in which a strong eugenic vision provided assurance that science and the right kind of gene (which was assumed to be primarily the possession of the white, educated, economically successful population) would ensure society's health, strength, and productivity. These eugenic assumptions were called into question by indications that cancer's rise not only existed "among civilized people living under better material conditions" but was actually more common among that population than those categorized as "primitive." This recognition added to the urgency of an approach that would offset the worrisome suggestion that the progress brought about by civilized society might be accompanied by health problems. Cancer rhetoric establishes a community of people who, although more susceptible to cancer by virtue of their privileges, were able to use their intelligence and resourcefulness to offset the dangers generated by the very civilization on which they had hung their hopes for social improvement.

Popular dissemination of cancer arguments reflected the importance of the dynamic relationship between danger and control. One of the primary themes in early efforts to publicize cancer acknowledged its capacity to strike *anyone* at *any time*. For example, a fundraising appeal for Memorial Hospital (renamed the Memorial Sloan Kettering Cancer Center in 1960), published in the New York tabloid the *Mirror* on December 19, 1945, emphasizes the disease's overwhelming and pervasive power:

> Now, I don't know how many folks will be gathered around your gala Yule tree for celebration, but let me give you this back-straightener, which will make you sit up and shiver: ONE OUT OF EVERY NINE PERSONS ALIVE IN THE UNITED STATES TODAY IS DOOMED TO DIE OF CANCER.
>
> Just whose name is next on the deadly roll call is anybody's guess! She may be sitting opposite you this Dec. 25 for dinner, but doomed to be among the missing a year from now. Even adorable Johnnie playing with his bright new fire engine may not be around for next year's festivities, because cancer is killing many children—it is no respecter of age.[55]

Of course it is a reality that cancer can strike anyone, but the sensational approach of this article reflects the "horror, fear, pity, compassion, and avoidance" that Davis describes as central to the way in which disability is "regulated, rationalized, contained."[56] This establishes a cycle that reverses and extends the euthenic pattern Currell identifies: panic is sparked by the recognition of cancer as a ubiquitous and unpredictable presence even among those "who may be sitting opposite you this Dec. 25 for dinner." The alarming recognition of imminent danger is followed by arguments that create idealized responses that mitigate the threat: courage, positivity, prevention. While these topoi might offer some degree of comfort through the vision of a society progressing in its ability to manage danger, they also contribute to "intensified fears of further eugenic decay."[57] At the same time, even this alarming passage provides a degree of distance, as the reader is personally affected by cancer, but in the role of an onlooker at a party in which others are among the afflicted.

Thus, cancer topoi participated in a euthenic transformation in which "laissez-faire responses to life . . . were to be replaced by self-insight, self-planning, and self-control."[58] While the initial impetus behind cancer rhetoric entailed the beneficial medical goal of saving lives, the entrenchment of topoi emphasizing "self-insight, self-planning and self-control" also aimed to shape healthy mindsets that would contribute to social progress—an example of the confidence and anxiety found in early twentieth century depictions of the role of self-improvement in health. Currell describes "self-improvement formulas" as grounded in the view "that mental ability was comparable to physical recovery."[59] This euthenic link between mental and physical health can be found in lines of argument that emphasized a combative, cheerful, or proactive mindset as central to cancer detection and recovery. These topoi were situated in larger discourses that reflected ambivalence about society's capacity to achieve the eugenic vision of progress, but they nevertheless constructed a people with a mindset equipped to face down a fearsome threat to public health.

THE POWER OF PUBLICITY

Certainly there were benefits available through encouraging people to face the problem of cancer head on. A 1940 article titled "A Brave Story" exults over the diminished shame felt by "people with mental disease, tuberculosis, cancer, venereal disease," who are now finding that their "stigmata are gradually being replaced by intelligent understanding."[60] And it was clear to many people that the shame surrounding cancer in past generations had negatively affected the potential for patients to receive the treatment they needed. A 1945 account of

Memorial Hospital's history explicitly links the public's ignorance about cancer in the nineteenth century to its neglect of cancer patients: "The founders were obliged to build it in what then were the outskirts of the city because of public opposition to such an institution. The public had not then learned that cancer is not contagious, or infectious or hereditary . . . So they gave the cancer hospital as wide a berth as possible and classified it merely as a place to which those stricken with cancer went to die."[61] Public education about cancer and the commitment of civic leaders within and beyond the ASCC during the early decades of the twentieth century made it possible for patients to escape from the isolation brought about from the sense of dread the public felt toward the disease, but of course "intelligent understanding" does not easily overcome all traces of the fears that had given rise to the stigma in the first place.

In addition to the goal of promoting knowledge and understanding, cancer rhetoric served the purpose of generating funds to support research and treatment needed to address an intractable and complex disease. This goal reinforced the need to spark public interest, as the focus of cancer publicity expanded to encourage support for research funding. A catalyst in the transformation of cancer publicity came about through the efforts of businesswoman and philanthropist Mary Lasker, whose recognition of the need for greater support for cancer research led her to the ASCC. After determining that the organization's fundraising efforts were insufficient for engaging a broader public, Lasker worked with her husband, Lord & Thomas advertising executive Albert Lasker, to alter the ASCC's communication strategy through the use of sophisticated advertising principles to promote cancer awareness. This effort involved taking on the challenge of balancing the organization's medical focus with the goal of public accessibility.[62]

During the same period, Sidney Farber, a cancer researcher at the Children's Hospital in Boston, was also exploring new strategies for increasing the visibility of cancer to generate public interest and funds for research. Farber's collaboration with Bill Koster of the Variety Club of New England led to the 1947 establishment of the Children's Cancer Research Fund, which developed a fundraising appeal centered on a young lymphoma patient named Einar Gustafson, who was given a new public identity of Jimmy, the poster child for the cause of children's cancer research.[63] Cancer biographer Siddhartha Mukherjee notes that the campaign's success taught Farber that "the campaign against cancer . . . needed icons, mascots, images, slogans—the strategies of advertising as much as the tools of science,"[64] an insight that shaped cancer advocacy in the decades following. In the late 1940s, Farber and Lasker became acquainted through their mutual ambition to heighten public awareness about cancer, and their aggressive emphasis on fundraising spread through the cancer community during this period.[65] While icons, mascots, images, and slogans helped bring cancer to life in ways that supported the goals of awareness and fundraising, these images also engaged the audience's fears in order to encourage support for research. But as noted previously, the incitement of fear as a motivating emotion, and the use of icons as images to fulfill the audience's obsessive need both to see and distance themselves from cancer, furthered the need to offer strategies for managing that fear through emphasizing the strength and control appropriate to members of a progressive society. These outlooks were offered through identification with cancer patients whose remarkable stories illustrated the attitudes suitable for overcoming the debilitating effects of cancer.

While the focus on hope provided a message that held positive benefits for cancer patients and the wider public, cancer rhetoric persistently reveals the fine line between the noteworthy goal of encouraging people not to despair at the prospect of cancer and the more problematic tendency to suppress the challenges that surround the experience of cancer diagnosis and treatment, an approach that parallels what Simi Linton describes as an effort to gloss over the embodied experiences of people with disabilities, serving "to mask the behaviors that would disturb the public and certainly not to exaggerate or call attention to our odd forms or the way our forms function."[66] While these messages likely encouraged public interest, iconic images of cancer patients also provided readers with a comforting "sense of normalcy," and an assurance that education and action entailed a measure of control.[67] A 1940 *New York Post* article supplements the 1936–39 statistics about Memorial Hospital patients with a look at "the figures that go down 68th St., to find hope and help." The story describes "a mother, her gray hair brushed up from too-flushed cheeks, neat and tidy under a matron's hat," who went without her family's knowledge to Memorial Hospital to investigate the pain in her left breast. The story suggests that readers should follow the woman's example in seeking expert advice in similar circumstances: "Well, she was scared, but not too scared to face facts. And she was taking care of it on time."[68] This portrait of the woman, "neat and tidy under a matron's hat," who took control of her destiny exemplifies Tasha N. Dubriwny's argument about the ways in which discourses that apparently empower women often feature narratives that confine them to the domestic sphere while pressing them to address significant public health issues. Like the women imagined in the "Go Red" campaign for women's heart health that is

Dubriwny's focus, the woman "who was not too scared to face facts" illustrates a central problem in medical rhetoric: "The promise of collective action is contradicted by an overall focus on the individual woman's responsibility to take care of her own health."[69]

What Dubriwny refers to as the "vulnerable empowered woman" has an important place in early cancer rhetoric. Likewise, children are also prominent figures who serve as poignant reminders of cancer's unpredictability. One highly publicized case was that of Charlie Hale, a three-year-old whose treatment for bone cancer at Memorial Hospital required the amputation of one leg. On January 7, 1946, newspapers across the country published emotionally charged articles about Hale, featuring titles that reveal a wide range of appeals. One cluster is primarily informative, such as the *Elizabeth Daily Journal* article titled, "Children's Cancer Real Challenge."[70] Others invoked pity through focusing on the child's inability to grasp what had happened to him, a response that reflected the adult reader's likely sense of the injustice that a child should have to face such a situation: "Three-Year-Old Cancer Victim Wonders When Docs Will Fix Leg and Bring It Back to Him"; "They Let Charlie Keep Thinking He'll Get His Leg Back—For They Know He Won't Live."[71] Others make a direct connection between the tragedy of Charlie's story and the need for additional funds for cancer research: "Dying Rutherford Lad's Parents Support Cancer Center Drive."[72] While these appeals adopted different perspectives, they collectively represented Hale in a way that managed the discomfort of cancer through pity, an emotion that assured readers that they were in touch with Hale's suffering. At the same time, Hale served as a mascot whose visibility and representation in sensationalized news stories provided a degree of distance from the complex reality of his experience.

Stories about children with cancer highlight the blurred lines between the nineteenth-century stigma toward people with cancer and the twentieth-century commitment to visibility. As Erving Goffman notes, the removal of social stigma often includes the tacit agreement that those who have been stigmatized will minimize the inconvenience that their visibility might cause to others by demonstrating their ability to adjust to conditions that others might find uncomfortable: "The nature of a 'good adjustment' . . . requires that the stigmatized individual cheerfully and unself-consciously accept himself as essentially the same as normals, while at the same time he voluntarily withholds himself from those situations in which normals would find it difficult to give lip service to their similar acceptance of him."[73] While his youth both heightened the audience's pity and made it impossible for Charlie Hale to offer reassurance by deliberately cultivating the strength and courage idealized in cancer topoi, his failure to understand the harsh reality of his prognosis in some respects lends itself to the "good adjustment" that Goffman notes. While it is surely a terrible thing to recognize that a child of three will not survive his disease, there is a degree of comfort in the fact that he continues to imagine himself as normal. As troubling as the prospect of cancer's capacity to strike children might be, in a strange and subtle way, the child's determination to sustain his usual activities aligns with the eugenic vision of social improvement that is sustained without interference from disability or disease. In some ways, children are ideal mascots for cancer rhetoric, not only because their stories prompt the emotional response that simultaneously creates passionate interest and a degree of detachment but also because the resilience of children serves as a useful exemplar in the construction of a people capable of maintaining a norm protected from the disruption of cancer.

Of course, the resilience of any cancer patient can be seen as cause for celebration, and the attention drawn to cancer through human interest stories, which seem particularly compelling when they depict the experiences of children, have historically held benefits including early detection and medical fundraising. At the same time, the circulation of such images evokes feelings that are inevitably complex, as are the cultural perspectives that solidify around such images. The use of mascots is fraught with ethical complications, as the intensity of the lived experience of those holding these roles may well be subsumed by the larger goals of communicating particular messages to the public. These messages often alleviate anxiety through illustrating what Dolmage describes as the "overcoming myth" in which people focus on the ability of remarkable individuals to overcome the challenges they face through tremendous skill or effort.[74] Dolmage goes on to note that this rhetorical trope functions "as a management of the fears of the temporarily able-bodied (if and when I become disabled, I will compensate or overcome), and it acts as a demand placed upon disabled people (you had better be very good at something)."[75] During this historical moment, the image of overcoming is also intricately woven into a tapestry of euthenic and eugenic discourses that simultaneously elevate and suppress the harsh reality of cancer in pursuit of a new social order attainable through partnership between science and those individuals capable of cultivating qualities that maximize their potential to achieve strength and resilience.

The effort to motivate the public's engagement with cancer generated rhetorical strategies that often departed from the goals of scientists, as reflected in a letter of protest from Frank Horsfall, president and director of Sloan Kettering

Institute, to John Heller, president of Memorial Sloan Kettering Cancer Center, after Horsfall's review of the draft of an NBC television script titled "Cancer Virus": "The thing is written with the obvious intent to excite and maintain audience interest. . . . This is the well-known Madison Avenue trick of utilizing interest in an important human problem to develop a huge viewing audience for the purposes of commercial backers rather than the transmission of accurate and appropriate scientific information."[76] Horsfall's rebuke reveals the problems that arise as cancer rhetoric circulates in new contexts that shape the ways in which cancer is represented. In a similar vein, the headline "Read This and Shiver" reflects the ways in which the effort to overcome the fear of cancer based in silence ironically circles back to tactics that reinscribe the fear and dread of an earlier era.[77] These tensions continued to be evident as the century progressed and strategies for marketing cancer became increasingly sophisticated.

INVISIBLE VISIBILITY

Cancer rhetoric consistently reflects the challenge of demonstrating confidence in the medical mastery of cancer without duplicating the nineteenth-century pattern of repulsion, which Davis describes as "a socially conditioned, politically generated response" toward people with disabilities.[78] The effort to challenge the silence about cancer through making the disease visible has the potential to unleash impulses to control that often follow awareness of disease: "If the norm regulates society by creating equal bodies, then medical theory, following suit, defines disease as a lack of regulation, an excess, that must be returned to a silent norm."[79] Cancer rhetoric's history reveals that, despite systematic efforts to remove it from the shadows, efforts to bring the disease into the public view are fraught, as the complex emotions surrounding cancer are managed by the use of icons, mascots, and images. As Susan Sontag notes, the metaphorical displacement of cancer from the materiality faced by people who have the disease reflects "the large insufficiencies of this culture: for our shallow attitude toward death, for our anxieties about feeling, for our reckless improvident responses to our real 'problems of growth,' for our inability to construct an advanced industrial society that properly regulates consumption, and for our justified fears of the increasingly violent course of history."[80] One inherent challenge of cancer rhetoric lies in the tension that emerges as the goal of imparting scientific information about a critical public health concern can only be achieved through making that information accessible to a public resistant to troubling images of debilitating weakness. The challenge of balancing vulnerability and strength, vigilance and progress, accounts for what at times appear to be conflicting messages in the inception of cancer rhetoric in the early decades of the twentieth century, and these patterns provide the foundation for topoi that have proven to have remarkable staying power.

2

Battling Cancer

HEROISM AND EUGENICS

The previous chapter discussed the ways in which the shift from silence to publicity in cancer rhetoric supported the formation of a people who were not only aware of cancer as a public health threat but also prepared to respond in ways that reflected and reinforced powerful cultural views about public health. While central assumptions about the desirable response of individuals who are ill remained fairly consistent across decades of the twentieth century, specific features of the topoi that construct this response shifted in ways that reflected the material conditions of particular historical moments. Throughout cancer rhetoric's evolution, however, central topoi collectively reinscribed the eugenic vision of progress that overcame the dangers a disease such as cancer posed to a thriving and robust populace.

Given the turmoil surrounding the period in which cancer became prominently featured in public discourse, it is unsurprising that an early topos in cancer rhetoric would be centered in metaphorical representations of cancer as an enemy and cancer treatment as a war. Many scholars have noted the importance of metaphor as a major trope of cancer rhetoric, as well as other public health rhetorics. Ulrich Teucher notes that metaphor's capacity to "suggest some kind of similarity between dissimilar terms" facilitates its role in difficult moments in which "people struggle to find words and explain a reality that seems to escape literal language."[1] Judy Segal's assessment of the importance of metaphor in medicine includes the recognition that "a study of biomedical metaphors should be a feature of the health policy debate."[2] At the same time, scholars such as Jackie Stacey argue that the tendency to rely on metaphor is particularly evident in the case of cancer.[3] Teucher concurs, as he situates the recognition that "cancer discourse abounds with metaphor" within a larger project of exploring the "struggle for meaning that appears to be particularly crucial in cancer."[4]

The strong link between metaphor and disease has not been without controversy. Susan Sontag's 1978 *Illness as Metaphor* offers a groundbreaking reflection on the vexed relationship between cancer and metaphor. Sontag argues that metaphorical language about diseases such as cancer and tuberculosis often creates "punitive or sentimental fantasies about that situation" that reflect "stereotypes of national character."[5] Sontag's stated aim in considering the relationship between metaphor and disease is to strip away the trappings of language that, she argues, diminish awareness of the disease's reality as an embodied phenomenon: "My point is that illness is *not* a metaphor, and that the most truthful way of regarding illness—and the healthiest way of being ill—is one most purified of, most resistant to, metaphoric thinking."[6]

Sontag makes a compelling case for the ways in which "metaphoric thinking" can detract from the cancer patient's lived experience of the disease. However, recent work across disciplines supports an interrogation of the division between metaphor and reality, offering a perspective that counters the apparent opposition between language about cancer and the "most truthful way" of capturing the embodied experience of illness. Jeanne Fahnestock's comprehensive view of the use of rhetorical figures in scientific rhetoric begins with the premise that the extensive focus on metaphor has at times limited attention to other figures, but she acknowledges that scientific metaphors are "numerous and compelling."[7] George Lakoff and Mark Johnson point out that metaphors play a central role in how people interpret their experiences; in fact, metaphors "govern our everyday functioning, down to the most mundane details," which connects with Sonja K. Foss's description of metaphor as offering a "way of knowing the world." Kenneth Burke notes the inescapability of metaphor in science and human life more generally: "Those who have criticized the use of metaphor have for the most part not realized how little removed such description is from the ordinary intellectual method of analysis."[8]

Their capacity to "govern our everyday functioning" helps to account for the fact that cancer metaphors constitute much of the public's relationship with cancer. In addition to shaping our understanding of ourselves in relation to the world around us, metaphors shape the public's imagination concerning what is possible. Stacey argues that metaphor cannot be separated from any aspect of medicine: "It is not only the experience of the illness that inevitably occurs in the domain of the metaphorical, but scientific and medical knowledge itself which is constituted according to certain metaphorical conventions."[9]

Segal concurs that the relationship between metaphor and science has material consequences, noting that "since biomedicine supplies the terms in which the health policy debate takes place, its metaphors act not only on medicine as it is, but also on medicine as it will be."[10] As is the case with other cancer topoi, metaphor not only shapes perceptions, attitudes, and decisions pertaining to health but also necessarily derives from the interactions of a network of diverse human and nonhuman actors. The significance of cancer metaphors can be grasped most fully through attending to the ways in which they acquire legitimacy through their connection to scientific developments and material conditions while establishing new frameworks for interpreting and responding to cancer as a threat to public health.

Thus, metaphors do not function solely as bridges between language and human experiences with cancer. Segal argues that the "biomedical model is not perpetuated by disengaged medical metaphors, but by a complex of forces, including a range of material ones."[11] Metaphors not only develop from the efforts of patients, health practitioners, and medical researchers to capture the nature of their experiences with the disease but also emerge from the reality constituted by the range of activities that cancer generates within a larger social context.

The materiality of metaphor and the relationship between social context and medicine is particularly evident in the connection between cancer and war. Although cancer rhetoric features a variety of metaphors, Segal identifies war as a central metaphor that runs through western biomedical discourse, while Teucher specifically identifies the dominance of the war metaphor in "the language of cancer."[12] These views are amply borne out by a historical study of cancer rhetoric, which reveals that the metaphorical connection with warfare persists across substantial changes in medical views of cancer and in larger cultural discourses during the twentieth century. In the discussion that follows, I argue that war metaphors can be more fully understood through a kairology that illuminates subtle shifts that take place as those metaphors circulate in different historical moments. Across their various formulations, these metaphors persistently establish frameworks that displace the threat to the vitality of modern society onto an external enemy that needs to be conquered through fortitude. While the mysterious mutation of healthy cells into cancerous ones happens internally, the resulting abnormality and its debilitating effects pose a threat not only to the body of the individual but also to the modern public's vision of the control available to people who demonstrate appropriate discipline and intelligence. The metaphor of cancer as enemy offers a eugenic displacement of a problem that can still be vanquished through a more concerted focus on the qualities of strength, resilience, and self-reliance that are the keys to sustained social progress. While the personification of cancer as enemy assumes different forms across decades of the twentieth century, the call for a militant response consistently constructs a people who are capable of meeting the challenge of cancer with courage and determination. Such a dynamic also rhetorically diminishes the focus on the effects of radical treatments on the bodies of patients, since the the damage chemotherapy and radiation inflict on healthy cells can be understood as a secondary hazard in the fight against the true enemy.

DISEASE PERSONIFIED

The metaphor of cancer as war illustrates what Foss describes as "symbolic convergence," the "frequent mention of a theme, a narrative, or an analogy in a variety of messages in different contexts."[13] Complex ecological factors in the United States coalesce in the symbolic convergence of the cancer battleground across the early decades of the twentieth century. These factors include historical and social developments that required the persuasive use of language to inspire public support for cancer research, treatment, and prevention; the significant role of the military in cancer research, including a persistent link between war weapons and evolving cancer treatments; and the intricate relationships among science, industry, the military, and medicine. An additional influence on the image of cancer as a battle was the emerging awareness of the character of cancer itself, which was persistently juxtaposed with the rhetorical formation of a people empowered to defeat cancer along with other threats to prosperity, social improvement, and democracy.

Although cancer was largely treated with silence prior to the twentieth century, the perception of cancer as a personified enemy has roots in the nineteenth century. Medical historian James P. Patterson describes cancer as maintaining a unique "hold on the popular imagination" during that period, the result of an intense dread of an "alien and living invader." According to Patterson, this image created a situation in which "people imagined cancers to be living moving creatures in themselves—uninvited beasts which surreptitiously ganged up on the body."[14] The notion of cancer as battle therefore has its roots in this period, even as limitations in medical knowledge and treatment options contributed to the general assumption that fighting against such a mysterious invader would be futile.

The rise of public cancer rhetoric in the twentieth century reflected a modern determination to assert the power of science and industry to resolve social problems, a spirit that was manifested in confidence in the benefits of early detection and treatment. During this period, war metaphors were deployed as an aggressive challenge to ignorance and to encourage people to pursue cancer testing that at that time represented the primary hope for saving lives. In 1927 the American Society for the Control of Cancer adopted "Fight Cancer with Knowledge" as its official slogan, making this idea visible on posters that featured images of St. George slaying the dragon of cancer.[15] In 1936 Clarence C. Little led the ASCC in establishing the Women's Field Army, which used the ranks, structure, and discipline associated with military life to recruit middle-class women for a campaign to educate the public about cancer.[16]

At the same time, an accompanying objective of public cancer rhetoric was to create a people whose response to public health crises would align with a broader national challenge to threats to American strength and prosperity. One step in the pursuit of this goal was to inspire the resolve that would encourage people to summon all available resources to combat cancer. One means of achieving this goal involved highlighting the mysterious and elusive character of this disease, a dangerous enemy capable of resisting the sophisticated advances in modern medicine that had successfully conquered other menaces to public health. The rising awareness of the facts surrounding cancer's invasion of human cells during the early twentieth century furthered the image of cancer as an intimate personal enemy and lent urgency to the notion of cancer as a battle that must engage the concerted efforts of cancer researchers, doctors, patients, families, and the general public. Such appeals emphasized the determined response necessary because of cancer's aggressive, unpredictable nature.

Depictions of this personified enemy repeatedly focused upon parallels between the behavior of cancer as a disease and the conduct of human villains who threaten the public's well-being. These depictions consistently reflect changing views of the ultimate threat to society at specific moments in history, which in turn shapes the type of war that must be waged to combat the enemy. The war against cancer in a 1942 *New York Journal-American* story reflects the mid-twentieth-century preoccupation with organized crime. The text of the article, titled "New Scientific Facts about Cancer—Chemicals That Strangle the 'Mad-Dog' Cells, Food Elements That Fortify the Body against their Ravages, Early Diagnosis and Other Advances in the Ceaseless Fight against Man's Worst Medical Enemy," updates and personifies the nineteenth-century view of the "uninvited beasts" of cancer that "ganged up on the body;" in this mid-twentieth-century US publication, cancer morphs into an actual gangster who points at a cowering man with an evil grimace. The accompanying article promises "good news from the battlefront" and goes on to say that, just as "crime is a cancer on the face of society," the converse side of that relationship is also true, for "cancer cells are wild, gangster cells in the human body that are 'outside the law.'"[17] The gangster metaphor provides the foundation for the article's description of the methods of cancer treatment available at that time: parole (ineffective), life imprisonment (radiation), and the death penalty (surgical removal).

In addition to the culturally scripted notion of the gangster as a pervasive and insidious enemy, the drawing accompanying the article contains another image that links the battle against cancer to eugenic views of disease as an encroachment on social goals that include racial purity as well as scientific and economic progress. The appearance of the gangster exaggerates stereotypical features associated with Jewish people: the nose, hair, and facial structure could well have signaled to the American reader of the 1940s an enemy that combined the widespread fear of both the underworld and the Jewish Other.[18] In her article discussing three studies of antisemitism in the United States during the 1940s, Eva-Maria Ziege notes that Pearl Harbor and the nation's 1941 entry into World War II heightened prejudice against various ethnic groups in the United States during the 1940s. Ziege states that "antisemitic violence was also a part of everyday life in the United States between 1941 and 1944"—the period of the article's publication. Ziege cites an American Jewish Committee poll that reflects a steady escalation in the percentage of Americans who perceived Jews as too powerful, rising from one-third in 1938–41 to 67 percent in 1945.[19] Given the widespread perception of Jews as a national threat during the period in which the article was published, it is not surprising that the threat of cancer might crystallize in an image that potentially not only reflected the public fear of gangsters but also located the threat of cancer as one component of larger anxieties that linked disease, social decay, and racial and ethnic purity.

At the same time, this period featured public awareness of an external enemy who posed an even greater threat to the strength of the nation. The menace of Hitler and the feeling of powerlessness sparked by Axis aggression were central to American consciousness before, during, and in the years following World War II. Images pertaining to Hitler and German aggression served as the basis for varying metaphorical representations of the evil of cancer. In an undated press release from the late 1940s announcing General Foods chair Clarence Francis's role in the Memorial Cancer Center Fund campaign, Francis refers to cancer as "the Gestapo of the human body" that "works just as slyly and as cruelly as did Hitler's henchmen." This parallel provides the basis for Francis's assertion that advances in cancer research are possible; although cancer "imposes as much torture on its helpless victims as Hitler and all his gauleiters combined," he insists that "it is we, the people, who decided that Hitler must go, and he went. Let us decide that cancer must go; let us pursue it as relentlessly as we pursued him."[20] Harry Schoenfeld, the head of that campaign's Women's Apparel Section, echoes the comparison between cancer and Hitler, adding, "We were thankful that the war against fascism is over, but we cannot feel secure as long as one disease, cancer, kills more than 160,000 persons a year in the United States alone."[21]

Other 1940s sources offer alternative images to support the argument for an aggressive attack against cancer. A 1945 *New York Post* article emphasizes cancer's wide reach: "This enemy shows no favoritism to any race, color, or creed. . . . It is the 'Fifth' Horseman—and when he runs amuck, incalculable suffering and tragedy follow. The Fifth Horseman is Cancer."[22] On occasion, journalistic shorthand provides the disease with nicknames that personify its danger, as in the 1946 *Dayton Daily News* article that describes research initiatives against "Killer Cancer."[23] Each metaphorical turn in these examples illustrates how persistent personifications of cancer—criminal, gangster, Hitler, Fifth Horseman, Killer—emerge from the disease's observed behaviors and reflect particular material concerns of the historical moments within which these discourses are situated. At the same time, each representation of the threat of cancer reflects the rhetorical strategy of summoning the audience to claim its rightful place as part of a people who are prepared to assert their national identity of strength and resilience in the face of all threats.

CANCER RESEARCHERS AT WAR

The image of the "death penalty" against gangster cancer cells, together with the notion that the national zeal against Hitler should be deployed against cancer, demonstrates how the broad rhetorical framework of cancer as battle was adapted to specific cultural contexts. Across early decades of the twentieth century, the two world wars influenced the development of battle metaphors that not only outlined an appropriate response for the public's encounter with the enemy of cancer but also constructed the battle faced by cancer researchers and clinicians. This line of argument shaped Curtis E. Lakeman's 1915 speech at a public meeting organized by the ASCC, which depicts the search for a cancer cure as a needed focus that offers an alternative to the current obsession with war but at the same time draws upon battle metaphors in describing cancer research:

> In this dark time which is passing like an eclipse across our once bright civilization, it is doubly necessary that we, in this country, should keep the torch of social progress burning, and strive for the ends of peace, so long as with honor we may. America has, indeed, no higher duty at the present time than to maintain one corner of earth where constructive efforts towards the alleviation of misery, the overthrow of injustice, the mitigation of poverty, and the prevention of disease can still be regarded as the chief end of the state.
>
> Among these ideals of peace none is more compelling than the conquest of the physical ills of mankind. Science holds out the fascinating prospect that if we will but follow the light of reason and effectively organize the social will and purpose, we can exterminate one after another of the great diseases, which afflict the race. A meeting like this devoted to thinking for an hour of such a glorious possibility should be in the highest degree a cheerful and inspiring occasion.
>
> But to bring the end of disease appreciably nearer we must all learn how to know the enemy and where to look for him.[24]

Lakeman's linking of the pursuit of peace to "the conquest of the physical ills of mankind" is significant, as is the insistence that science and "the light of reason" hold the key that will "organize the social will" in support of "the conquest of the physical ills of mankind." While the hope of protecting people from cancer is an admirable goal, the language of a national will to overcome health challenges resonates with eugenic ideologies.

The pursuit of a "conquest of the physical ills of mankind" as a form of war supporting the "ideals of peace" in cancer discourse continues during the World War II era. A headline circa 1940 refers to architectural developments at Memorial Hospital as a "New Battleground in Cancer War," while another 1940 article situates Memorial Hospital's cancer research within a battle that counters the destructive war taking place in Europe and provides greater assurance of the pursuit of modern advancement: "Memorial Hospital, in E. 68th St., surrounded by a world at war and bent on destruction, is a place where you actually can see progress on the march, in terms that can be measured, toward a finer civilization."[25] Lehigh University president Clement C. Williams elaborates this view in a 1940 speech to the New York Patent Law Association: "It would be an unnatural atavism that could find a greater sense of natural pride and satisfaction in the crushing of Paderewski's Poland, pious and cultured Czechoslovakia, or valiant and honorable Finland, than in the discoveries of scientists, which have so blessed mankind."[26] The effort to explain the approach necessary for effective cancer treatment often includes war analogies, as in a 1946 *New York World-Telegram* article about the cancer detection efforts at the Strang Clinic of Memorial Hospital: "Treating active cancer is like trying to repel an enemy after he has invaded and destroyed part of your homeland. A better way—when it is possible—is to seek out any fifth column and eradicate it before the invasion is serious."[27]

At the same time, the relationship between war and cancer is not only metaphorical but is forged through material conditions that established a strong historical connection between war and cancer research and treatment. Daniel Sarewitz notes that many developments in modern science have come "not from 'the free play of free intellects,' but from the leashing of scientific creativity to the technological needs of the U.S. Department of Defense."[28] George J. Annas attributes the dominance of the military metaphor in part to the fact that "until recently, most U.S. physicians had served in the military;" indeed, the intersections between the medical community and the battlefield also account for the fact that many advances in cancer treatments originated in military research.[29] Surgery continued to be the dominant treatment during this period, but war brought new advances in surgery and increased the public's faith in its potential.[30] The link between cancer research and the military also helps to account for the number of gains in cancer research that took place in the years between the two world wars. The deployment of mustard gas in both conflicts advanced the use of chemotherapy for cancer treatment. Cornelius P. Rhoads, who was appointed director of Memorial Hospital in 1940, was also a medical officer in the US Army whose responsibilities included chemical weapons research, for which he received the War Department's Legion of Merit Award in 1945.[31] Siddhartha Mukherjee notes that Rhoads's appointment at Memorial facilitated "the connection between the chemical warfare of the battlefield and the chemical warfare of the body," a connection evident to the press of that era.[32] Rhoads appeared on the cover of a 1949 *Time* magazine cover that bore the caption, "Cancer-Fighter Cornelius P. Rhoads—Some Gangsters Are Vulnerable."[33]

The material connection between the field of oncology and the military, alongside the noticeably aggressive nature of the disease itself, helps to account for verbal representations of cancer treatments as weapons suited for battle. The 1939 *New York Post* announcement of the dedication of Memorial Hospital's new facility makes note of the hospital's purchase of an x-ray machine powered by $90,000,000 worth of radium, "a virtual arsenal of anticancer weapons."[34] Another article on the hospital's opening, titled "Dispatch from the Front," begins, "From front-line trenches of the war on cancer comes good news" and goes on to describe the hospital's million-volt x-ray machine as "a new and powerful war weapon."[35] Multiple headlines and articles from this period duplicate this image: "An unprecedented million-volt X-ray machine to probe healingly into the evil mysteries of deep malignant growths . . . is just one of the many scientific weapons with which the new Memorial Hospital for the Treatment of Cancer and Allied Diseases is equipped to combat mankind's number one enemy;" "New Hospital Wages Modern War on Cancer;" "Radium Moved across Town . . . Bomblike Leaden Container Is Guarded by Police."[36]

The development of "weapons" of treatment and the growth of major cancer centers during and immediately following World War II together underscore the pervasive material relationship between war and cancer, a relationship that sustains the dynamic connection between cultural preoccupations and emerging language and images of cancer during this period. Particularly during the early years of the war, the battle against cancer continued to be held up as a worthy enterprise that contrasted favorably with the necessity of fighting human evil. A widely circulated 1942 article compares the hope surrounding the war on cancer with what at that time seemed to be a more discouraging international landscape: "If this is a time when faith in mankind flags, when we doubt man's progress and question the worth of his spirit and his intellect, a digression from the news of war, man against man, to news of war, man against disease, will be restorative."[37] Optimism about the potential of chemotherapy provides an ongoing contrast with anxiety about war on the battlefield, as is evident in a 1943 *American Weekly* article: "Good news comes from the battlefront where medical science is attacking the problems of cancer. . . . Here is the last minute communiqué in this war against one of man's greatest killers! Chemicals are being discovered which attack, by strangulation, human cancer cells without doing an equal amount of harm to normal body tissues so far studied."[38] Subsequent developments disproved the expectation that chemotherapy would attack only harmful cells, but the assumption that cancer treatment could offer a scientific means for engaging people in a life-saving war against a common enemy is noteworthy.

The strong material and metaphorical ties between war and cancer research at times encouraged the view that the two were ideologically linked, through language that summoned a people prepared to battle cancer as an important component in the eugenic pursuit of the American vision of strength, prosperity, and social improvement. In an address at the 1939 Memorial Hospital dedication, former Cornell president Jacob Gould Schurman connects patriotic fervor, scientific progress, individual freedom, civilization, and cancer research:

> That is the danger today in not a few of the countries of Europe including some of the most populous and powerful. They have enthroned force above the free spirit of man. The precious and inalienable life of the individual has been subjugated and suppressed by dictatorial regimentation and control, which, within those nations, is as irresistible as it is universal and all-embracing.
>
> America is the land of freedom. Freedom has made our people what they are. I appeal to you to guard and maintain that freedom with whole-hearted loyalty and devotion.
>
> This lofty and massive structure, with its finely equipped hospital and laboratories, is itself a splendid monument to the spirit of freedom. It would not be here today, if in the former home of the hospital, intelligent founders and benefactors and competent scientific investigators had not been free to develop and apply their ideas.[39]

Schurman's depiction of the intrinsic link between science, freedom, and democracy is reflected in discourses that seamlessly connect confidence about the outcome of the war against the Axis powers with the war against cancer. One section of a 1942 New York Cancer Institute Social Service Auxiliary brochure detailing the social services available for cancer patients contains the slogan, "Our Hope—Victory in War—Victory over Cancer," bordered in alternating red V's with blue stars.[40]

The years following the war saw an explosion in research funding, which in turn generated an increase in medical knowledge, changes in medical education, and more focused specializations.[41] There was also a growing conviction among medical professionals that the insights acquired from the war could benefit cancer researchers in the future. A 1944 Memorial Hospital press release contains extensive quotes from a lecture titled "Cancer and the Public" by Clarence C. Little, who was at that time managing director of the ASCC, which emphasize the benefits of connecting cancer research to military strategy:

> As we proceed to do this, we shall find a direct and impressive parallel between the problems and conditions of actual warfare and those involved in the control of cancer. In any situation leading towards war there are to be found elements of insufficient knowledge of our potential adversary. Had the world understood the basic psychology of the Japanese people and their leaders, steps could have been taken in advance of Pearl Harbor to avert the type of war in which the initiative was left in the hands of the enemy. Deliberate or stupid ignorance is as evil in our fight against cancer as it has proven to be in our war on Japan. . . . We now find our allies and ourselves pledged to do the necessary international research in the motives of nations after the war—so that the origin of greed, aggression and domination by force can be detected and understood. In just the same way we find hundreds of men and women devoting their lives to the search for conditions and circumstances that lead to the origin of cancer.[42]

Little continues the extended analogy throughout the speech, demonstrating what for him are the material benefits of considering direct parallels between military strategy and cancer research.

This fusion continues to be evident in cancer treatments developed in the years following the end of World War II. In April 1946 Maj. Gen. Alden H. Waitt of the chemical warfare service announced new research linking mustard gas to leukemia treatment at a press conference held during the American Chemical Society's 109th meeting. Media coverage of this development was widespread, much of it focusing on the promise "that war research on chemical and bacteriological weapons had opened up new lines of humanitarian attacks against certain forms of cancer."[43] The increased use of radioactive materials for cancer testing is also traced to the war; although a September 1946 *Atlanta Journal* article acknowledges that the radioactive solution used to understand cancer's development is "not a byproduct of the atom bomb," the writer goes on to explain that recent developments in nuclear research have reduced the cost of the material and made it more accessible for the purposes of cancer research.[44] One headline announcing Memorial Hospital's receipt of an isotope called carbon 13, developed by Eastman Kodak, reads, "Hospital Gets First Atomic Weapon Today."[45]

The emergence of the military-industrial complex across the decades spanning the two world wars had a noticeable impact on cancer rhetoric. As early as 1940 the *New York Herald Tribune* signaled the pursuit of new ties among medicine, the military, and industry, citing Rhoads's view that "basic information and technical procedures" that could contribute to cancer research could be found immediately "in every laboratory of industrial chemistry."[46] The strong ties between science and corporate America that had bolstered eugenic rhetoric in the 1920s and 1930s continued to be evident in material support for cancer research and in rhetoric that connected advances in cancer treatment to national progress. Numerous initiatives in cancer research during the 1950s and 1960s featured a cooperative venture on the part of the military, industry, and medical researchers; for example, a 1953 letter to cancer philanthropist Mary Lasker from Edwin B. Wilson of the Office of Naval Research attributes the emergence of the ultraviolet color translating microscope to a partnership between the Office of Naval Research, Memorial Hospital, and Polaroid, along with support from the American Cancer Society (ACS).[47]

Such alliances infused cancer rhetoric with a new spirit of hopefulness during the postwar period, which included confidence in the power of industry and technology to control the nation's destiny. The *New York Times* touted Sloan-Kettering Institute, the new research branch of Memorial Hospital established in 1948 by General Motors executives Alfred P. Sloan and Charles F. Kettering, as "the first application of American industrial research techniques to cancer research."[48] The *Times* article announcing the facility's opening states that "the dramatic news of the atomic bomb, developed by a $2,000,000,000 research program, was a 'graphic illustration' of what can be accomplished by scientifically organized research as practiced by American industry. If as much money and talented personnel were available as the Government had had for the atomic bomb . . . 'very rapid' progress could be made in cancer research." In the same article, Sloan attests to the view that the "broad principles of organized industrial research" can provide the foundation for cancer breakthroughs.[49] The discovery of the benefits available through partnership with industry served as a catalyst for new models of cancer research that would carry forward into the latter decades of the twentieth century. In a speech at the opening of the Sloan-Kettering Institute, Federal Security Administrator Oscar Ewing builds on the shift from military engagement to an Institute aimed at the "conquest of cancer": "The relation of science to military preparedness is obvious. But scientific discovery is even more essential to progress against poverty and disease." Ewing emphasizes the relevance of insights gained from military research to cancer: "The experience of the last seven or eight years, in war and peace, has also taught us that scientists in and out of Government can work together in various ways, and that they must work together in those ways to achieve their common objectives."[50] In his contributions to a panel discussion featured at the Sloan-Kettering opening, Paul C. Aebersold, chief of the Atomic Energy Commission's Isotopes Division, applauds the rapid progress in science and technology, adding, "During the late war valuable lessons were learned and new patterns set for cooperation in research and development. The spectacular success of numerous war-time projects, not only in chemical and physical fields but in the medical field as well, demonstrated convincingly the great combination of creative and productive power that derives from close teamwork between universities, government, technology, and laymen—or in other terms between science, administration, industry, and the public."[51]

Numerous media articles from this period expressed modern confidence about the union of industrial research methods and medicine. Arguments pertaining to new research methods both shaped and reflected changing public perceptions about scientific authority and expertise. A *New York Sun* article stresses that the significance of the Sloan Foundation grant lies not in the size of the donation alone but in "the manner in which it is to be spent, a manner which issues a study of cancer that will employ the same broad, yet intensive, technical thoroughness which has wrought such wonders in industrial research."[52] An editorial in the *Santa Barbara News-Press* suggests that it is time to replace the "prima donna type of research long in favor" among scientists with the brilliant minds found in the corporate world, adding, "It is fair to assume that corporations which spend huge sums on research are not without geniuses and that these are happy enough when they work on an assigned project at a salary.... For the first time we shall see what organization, planning and competent direction can do in conquering a disease that now stands second in the list of causes of death."[53] However, a contrasting perspective is offered in numerous articles that highlight the importance of traditional research and caution the public against assuming that scientific breakthroughs come from an assembly of workers rather than intensive scientific research. One example, published in the *Monticello Evening News* (Monticello, New York), expresses concern that recent news coverage may have confused the public about the importance of fundamental cancer research: "Most of those writing about the atomic bomb mistakenly assumed that the public understood that the bomb development was possible only because fundamental discoveries made by widely separated scientists working on their own initiative were applied by scientists familiar with one or more of them and were willing to work together in the service of their country."[54]

Aebersold's example of the atomic project as the exemplar of "the astonishing success" possible through cooperation between science and industry provides a further link between the war against external human enemies and the war against cancer. Aebersold and other speakers insist that they are not suggesting that cancer research can precisely emulate the approach of the "wartime atomic energy project" or the methods of "an industrial research project."[55] However, the entwinement of war, medicine, and industry is less finely tuned as this relationship circulates through media accounts. A story in the *Phoenix Republic* contrasts the government investment in the atomic bomb with the more modest amount invested in the establishment of the Sloan-Kettering Center but adds, "Oddly, perhaps, it was explained that the release of energy which makes the atomic bomb so destructive may be utilized in the study of concer [*sic*] and its treatment. The atomic bomb may never be used again in warfare because wars may end, but the war against cancer is still going on and use of atomic energy in conquering it would be applauded."[56]

Many lines of argument in the media align cancer treatment even more closely with atomic weapons. An article in the *San Francisco News* simply states, "Fortunately there is a similarity between cancer research and the research which led to the atomic bomb."[57] The announcement of the Sloan-Kettering opening in the *Stamford Advocate* assures readers that "even the atomic bomb may have brought us nearer the answer to the age-old cancer question, for already 'artificial radioactive substances' have been used as radium substitutes in treating the disease."[58] The Memorial Cancer Center fund-raising radio spots of the late 1940s are more vague in alluding to the connections between cancer treatment and atomic weapons. A one-minute spot announcement begins with the reminder, "We stood toe to toe with three vicious Axis powers and won a costly war. There is a greater enemy still waging a dangerous war against us," while another notes, "The atom bomb was developed by bringing together the scientists who knew most about the atom, providing them with adequate help and materials and concentrating their combined knowledge on the problem. There is no lack of cancer specialists in America."[59] The announcement suggests that Memorial Cancer Center has the team in place to apply the collaborative strategies used in atomic research to address the problem at hand. While these announcements do not promise that the precise methods used in building the atomic bomb and defeating the Axis enemy will lead to such a decisive victory in the war against cancer, the public is encouraged to believe that the research methods that led to victory in one war could be useful in the pursuit of an enemy that has taken even more American lives.

Of course, the end of World War II meant heightened attention to an ally-turned-enemy, and this concern was reflected in cancer rhetoric as well. In a 1949 speech about Memorial Hospital's five-million-dollar expansion project, Edmund E. Day, chancellor of Cornell University, urges the public not to allow the distraction of communism to jeopardize the focus on cancer as the true enemy: "There is a tide in the affairs of men in which the cold war with Russia is but a dramatic surface storm. . . . The future belongs to those who know most . . . We must make our knowledge serve social ends. Here the Communists have us under a challenge. Let us make sure we meet this challenge to the hilt. We can, if we will, find what Henry James called the 'moral equivalent of war.' No engagement is more important than that being waged against cancer. Here is an enemy that is a scourge the world over."[60]

The fading memory of the world war across the ensuing decades facilitated a stronger focus on the war against the internal enemy and a shift in the ways in which the ever-resilient enemy of cancer was discursively represented. The end of the war created space for cancer activists to reflect on the disparity between the cost of military engagement as compared with the nobler war against cancer. After decades in which the fate of cancer research seemed to be inextricably entwined with the military, cancer activists began to recognize that the interests of the two were not in fact identical and to assert cancer as a priority in the competition for limited government resources. Even before the war ended, in a 1944 *New York Times* article, Fred W. Stewart, acting director of Memorial Hospital during Rhoads's military service, notes, "Deaths from cancer since Pearl Harbor have exceeded many times the deaths in combat in the armed forces of the United States."[61] In a 1948 article, Florida gubernatorial candidate Fuller Warren argues for greater attention to cancer research, even as he explicitly avoids criticizing the vast sums that had been spent on the development of the atomic bomb: "Most of us feel that the late President Roosevelt did a wise, humane thing when he authorized the expenditure of two billion dollars for the development of the atomic bomb. The bomb saved thousands of American lives which would have been lost if it had been necessary to invade Japan. But when we contrast the niggardly $12,544,000 for cancer research with the staggering $2,000,000,000 for the A-bomb, we realize that Congress is being shortsighted indeed."[62]

The long-standing pattern of linking cancer and war persisted in the decades following World War II, while the rhetorical construction of cancer, cancer treatments, and war continued to reflect new insights about cancer shaped by emerging cultural anxieties. Arguments for federal support for cancer research in the 1950s and 1960s reflected efforts to sustain public optimism about the potential of scientific research. Accompanying a 1966 *Life* magazine feature article titled "The All-Out Assault on Leukemia," Albert Rosenfeld offers "A Superplan to Cut Years Off the War," featuring a flow chart that demonstrates the use of "Convergence Technique," which Rosenfeld explains is "designed to make hundreds of separate projects converge toward a single purpose—the control and cure of leukemia—in the same highly organized way the Manhattan Project set out to produce an A-bomb."[63] Rosenfeld's full explanation of the link between cancer research and atomic production captures an idea that is frequently referenced in the concise phrase "Manhattan Project for cancer" during this period. The persistent metaphor "magic bullet" to connote an effective medical treatment is used to describe chemotherapy in a 1956 American Cancer Society pamphlet.[64] Thus, the image of chemotherapy as weapon is fused with the fact of its development in war laboratories and its metaphorical representation as the counter to cancer, the resilient and personal enemy. At the same time, new realities in the American experience of war facilitated new ways of capturing key features of humanity's encounter with cancer, such as Stanford biologist Donald Kennedy's description of cancer in the 1960s as a "medical Vietnam."[65]

The persistent pattern of juxtaposing the large investment in the military with the limited resources available for medical causes escalated in the latter decades of the century. Richard Nixon's declaration of war on cancer in 1971 appeared to hold great promise, but it quickly became apparent to cancer advocates that other wars were being given preference over cancer research. An Ann Landers column in 1971 laments the fact that "the lion's share of the tax dollar is going for defense," noting that "for every man, woman and child in the United States our government spent $125 on the war in Vietnam, $19 on the space program, $19 on foreign aid, 89 cents on cancer research."[66] Two years later, a *Washington Post* article addressing the disappointing outcome of

President Nixon's pledge to combat cancer places much of the blame on defense spending; Warren Magnuson, chair of the health appropriations subcommittee, notes that "the cost of the secret bombing raids in Cambodia—$140 million—is the same as the money cut from the cancer program's request."[67] In 1974 the *National Observer* described the war on cancer as "an effort that could prove to be medicine's own Hundred Years' War," pointing to controversies among scientists about the premature nature of the crusade and the potential of a concerted emphasis on cancer to damage other health initiatives.[68] Such struggles over resources underscore the complex ways in which the ecological relationships among cancer, medical treatments, the military, and public resources are rhetorically enacted.

THE COMPLEXITY OF CANCER METAPHORS

The persistent depiction of cancer as war reflects shifting cultural perspectives across time. While the verbal and visual depictions of the enemy shift in ways that resonate with emerging historical events, the overarching goals of courage, strength, and resilience are constant. As discussed previously, the notions of cancer as an enemy and treatment as battle reflect material conditions surrounding cancer research and treatment, and they also resonate with the experiences of many people with cancer. At the same time, the repeated use of this topos also demonstrates cancer rhetoric's imbrication in broader cultural discourses that are shaped by eugenic imperatives concerning social improvement and progress. These areas of emphasis often work against the empowerment they appear to promise, since they suppress the complexity of individual experience through an emphasis on a singular narrative of power that overcomes challenges. In "Breast Cancer Narratives as Public Rhetoric: Genre Itself and the Maintenance of Ignorance," Judy Segal claims that the formulaic character of the genre of breast cancer narratives contributes to public ignorance about cancer, as these stories "suppress or replace other genres in which breast cancer might be queried and explored."[69] The same can be said of war metaphors, whose dominance in public life and material presence in the medical community structure the options available to people in responding to cancer. Just as Ceccarelli points to the hidden violence embedded in the vision of science as conquering the frontier, the war metaphor and the personification of cancer as a sinister external enemy sometimes obscure the fact that cancer patients are dealing with a disease that has emerged from within their own cells. In her incisive critique of the representation and treatment of cancer,

Azra Raza asks, "How do we define this war when the body has to shield itself from internal and external aggressions simultaneously? It is a war for the body, on the body, by the body. The patient, held hostage by inside and outside forces, becomes aware of parts they never knew existed until unbearable pain and inflammation or a popping tumor or damage by chemotherapy unceremoniously bring them into the conscious realm."[70] The public obsession with the war metaphor illustrates what Kristen Lindgren describes as a false opposition between the purity of self and the corruption of disease. Drawing on anthropologist Emily Martin's study of the representation of the immune system, Lindgren argues that both metaphors of warfare and of the body as a police state suggest that "the protection and solidification of self-identity is central."[71] Given that the nature of disease leads to "the breakdown of the clear boundary between self and other, inside and outside," Lindgren suggests that "it is necessary to rethink the structure of selfhood," a call that Sontag anticipates in characterizing the cancer war metaphor as "implicitly genocidal."[72] The genocidal function of the war metaphor provides a striking example of Henri-Jacques Stiker's "fear of the abnormal" that leads to "the desire to kill."[73]

While the desire to destroy cancer is shared by people with cancer and the general public, the process of creating a people capable of overpowering disease through strength of will connects with eugenic undertones that obscure difference through imposing the comforting pursuit of normalcy on every situation. One example can be found in the 1946 death of three-year-old Charles Hale from bone cancer referenced in chapter 1. Headlines repeatedly connected Hale's death with the war on cancer. For example, the *New York Herald Tribune* headline announces, "A Child's Death Spurs the War against Cancer," a view echoed by the *New York Times*: "Boy's Death Spurs Fight on Cancer."[74] The assumption of cancer as a battle also constructs the patient as the hero of that battle, as illustrated in the *New York Journal-American* headline, "Heroic Lad of 3 Dies of Cancer."[75] In drawing attention to these headlines, I am by no means questioning the character of Charles Hale and his family, but I am pointing to the ways in which powerful metaphors function in cases such as this to subsume the lived experiences of individuals within a larger narrative that supports the cultural value of strength that draws attention away from the debilitating effects of illness. In her incisive analysis of a news story describing a three-year-old leukemia patient as a "true fighter who never gave in to her disease," Segal writes, "the description deposits on the child the anxieties of adults in the grip of a metaphor they have forgotten is a metaphor, betraying everyone's lack of narrative imagination."[76] The child who is a determined fighter provides an anxious public with an image that makes cancer more visible and emotionally fraught, but at the same time creates an emotional distance through focusing on disembodied courage that offers stability and hope that surpasses the uncertainty of an individual's health crisis.

Many examples demonstrate the "grip" of the war metaphor in ways that have direct consequences for the public's perception of the experience of cancer and cancer patients' understanding of the responses they are encouraged to adopt. As Sontag notes, even the most brutal treatment must be accepted bravely by cancer patients aware that they are engaged in battle. The scope of this narrative dictates that "there can be no question of pampering the patient."[77] Within the complex narrative of the battle between self and disease, Sontag argues, "Ostensibly, the illness is the culprit. But it is also the cancer patient who is made culpable."[78] A. Suresh Canagarajah explicitly engages with this problem in describing his feelings about the well-meaning advice of friends following a cancer diagnosis: "They said they were praying that I should win this battle, like the other challenges I had overcome in the past. This metaphor of battle has been in American public discourse since the 'war on cancer' slogan by President Nixon in the 1970s. However, the metaphor filled me with dread. If I die, would my relatives say that I didn't fight hard enough or that God had abandoned me? While some blamed me for causing the disease, might others blame me for succumbing to it? I wouldn't come out of these judgments looking good either way, I thought to myself."[79] Even if cancer patients who are unable to be victorious in battle are not directly blamed for the outcome of a disease they cannot control, the war metaphor imposes the expectation that those who have violated the standards of normality that are so vital to the health of society can redeem the situation through a courageous response, a posture that sustains the eugenic emphasis on the alliance between science and strength of will.[80] While it might be impossible for cancer patients to avoid what Bernarr Macfadden considered the "sin" of sickness, cancer rhetoric centered in the topoi of war and battle ensure that cancer patients need not succumb to the "crime" of "weakness."[81]

In addition to constructing a people focused on strength and resilience, cancer topoi influence how people with cancer understand their experience. Stacey writes, "My experience of cancer was circumscribed by this powerful (and potentially very persuasive) 'textual body' of discourse which draws upon some centrally shared, and increasingly common-sense, cultural beliefs."[82] She argues that representations of cancer are characterized by "the desire for order and control" based in "a masculine drive to mark out the boundaries of a separate territory."[83] Kristen Garrison explores the consequences of the war metaphor's ubiquity for women diagnosed with breast cancer; although she acknowledges that this image may be useful for some women, Garrison argues for the need to pursue alternative rhetorical frameworks that offer people dealing with illness and disability a wider range of narrative options.[84]

Yet the zeal for control reflects an impulse to define Western medicine in terms that align with battle terminology and that emphasize victory above all, an image that squarely situates cancer patients in a realm of internal tension. Segal notes that "biomedicine in general has not been able to articulate a place for death as anything other than defeat or failure" and adds that the wins and losses of metaphorical wars against disease indirectly establish "a field of combat in which it is increasingly difficult to identify the enemy."[85] Teston argues that the lines of argument that personify cancer as "the enemy" ultimately "promulgate militaristic paradigms that vilify bodies."[86] Given that the cancer war frequently entails the view that "cancer is the *self* at war with the *self*," the ultimate outcome of an unsuccessful battle may assume that the "person as medical failure is the enemy."[87] And according to the principles of eugenic thought, this is the case, since any unresolved threat to the norm must be displaced for the sake of society's untroubled advancement.

In addition to the complications that the war metaphor creates for cancer patients, there are negative consequences of accepting without question the historical links between cancer research and the military-industrial complex. Like other such metaphors—the war on drugs, the war on crime, the war on poverty—cancer research and war are separate endeavors, and to confuse the two risks diminishing the attention and respect given to medical concerns that are distinct from the methods and aims of the military. History tells us that when it was necessary to make the choice between Cambodian bombing raids and the funding allocations for the war on cancer, the physical war was given precedence over the metaphorical one.

Yet the recognition that a metaphor is problematic does not readily eradicate it from popular use. One issue is that the war metaphor is not entirely negative. Teucher acknowledges that the war metaphor is "divisive" but also notes that it is "rousing and gives voice to the anger that one feels, and it provides a focus for one's energies in times of chaos."[88] Moreover, metaphor is not easily removed from public life through focused initiatives. Segal expresses appreciation for the concerns Annas raises in insisting that problematic verbal images, including the military metaphor, should be displaced from health care debates;

however, she recognizes the difficulty of controlling metaphors that are so intricately woven into cultural discourses.[89]

I concur with Segal's view that language about cancer is too complex to be externally managed. At the same time, cancer rhetoric will continue to evolve alongside the material conditions surrounding the disease and its treatment, since language is always embedded in culture. Insights of scholars such as Lindgren, Raza, and Stacey that complicate the oppositions between self and disease, changing public attitudes toward warfare, new insights about the nature and causes of cancer, and shifting relations between the medical community and the military industry will likely alter the salience of the war metaphor over time. Perhaps even more significant will be recent changes in cancer treatment that emphasize the goal of keeping the disease in check rather than total annihilation, which may well generate new representations of cancer and its relationship with the human body. However, the anxiety that drives rhetorics about disease, as well as disability, must be under constant scrutiny, since that anxiety often blends seamlessly with eugenic assurances that violently reinscribe the power of an elusive norm in order to provide reassurance that progress can be maintained in spite of evidence to the contrary. The recognition of the intricate interconnections among language, disease, culture, and the embodied experiences of patients offers useful insight into the complexity surrounding both past and emerging cancer rhetorics—and serves as an important reminder of the need to attend to the power of discourse to exclude the bodies, identities, and experiences of those who are unable to accommodate themselves to a long-standing cultural ideal.

3

Thinking Positive

PROGRESSING BEYOND CANCER

My husband and I sat side by side in the waiting room on the day of his first appointment at the oncology center. On the wall opposite us was a large poster advertising "Camp Good Days and Special Times," a local program offering support groups, arts and crafts workshops, and outdoor activities for cancer patients and their families. Behind us, a cancer patient sat between two women sporting halos, pink tutus and tights, and large pink wings, who informed the receptionist that they had designated themselves "good fairies" who would assume responsibility for livening up their friend's chemotherapy treatment. As we listened to the explosions of giggling behind us, my husband turned to me and commented, "It's hard to accept that I'm now part of a population that everyone is trying this hard to cheer up."

I have no way of knowing how the woman awaiting her chemotherapy treatment felt about her friends' desperate attempts to cheer her up, but I couldn't help wondering if she shared at least something of the feeling my husband expressed. What I also recognized was that this moment connects with a much larger network of cancer topoi emphasizing the importance of maintaining a cheerful and positive outlook that can be seen by others. The goal of "cheering people up" might on the surface appear to be unequivocally positive. However, this book invites the question of whether people with cancer are really the ones whose interests are served by urgings to manifest a positive disposition, or whether they instead might be seen as the unwitting catalysts for a eugenic impulse to assert that the cultivation of a healthy mental state can counter the debilitating effects of disease.

Many cancer patients have expressed frustration with the cultural pressure to adopt a happy disposition in circumstances where such an outlook does not appear to be warranted and in fact adds to their burden rather than diminishing it. One of the most well-known critiques of the culture of cheer in the contemporary cancer world can be found in the work of Barbara Ehrenreich, who challenges the assumption that positive thinking must be inherently beneficial, countering that "the sugar-coating of cancer can exact a dreadful cost."[1] She argues that the "tyranny of positive thinking" forces "the denial of understandable feelings of anger and fear, all of which must be buried under a cosmetic layer of cheer."[2] Although Ehrenreich acknowledges that cheerfulness might be the response that family, friends, and care providers hope for in cancer patients, she insists that this creates pressure that cannot be justified. Perhaps the most damaging indictment of the tyranny of positive thinking is evident in cases where treatment is unsuccessful, which according to Ehrenreich has the potential to leave the patient blaming the outcome of the disease on her own negativity.[3] Audre Lorde calls for a response to cancer that constitutes an "affirmation of self" distinct from "looking on the bright side of things," an outlook that she describes as "a euphemism used for obscuring certain realities of life, the open consideration of which might prove threatening or dangerous to the status quo."[4]

Despite these concerns, cancer topoi of positivity, like the topos of cancer as enemy, have a long history—one that intersects with disability and is inflected with eugenic ideologies concerning the management of conditions deemed abnormal. In discussing the period before society was expected to accommodate people with disabilities, Sharon L. Snyder and David T. Mitchell write, "Without the necessity of demands on accessible and flexible social environments, disabled people function almost exclusively as a lesson for the nondisabled, promoting behaviors such as patience, cheerfulness, and 'making the best of things.'"[5] As has been the case with people with disabilities, the insistence that people with debilitating illnesses must "make the best of things" may be framed as a positive outcome for them, but its actual function is arguably to offer inspiration to others, as well as a measure of reassuring distance from the problem. Above all, it protects those who frantically cling to their "mutual membership in the realm of the normal" from confronting the reality that a disease such as cancer "might prove threatening or dangerous to the status quo."[6]

The impulse to protect the status quo is evident in many arguments surrounding the benefits of positivity in responding to cancer. As is the case with war topoi, the topos of positivity emerged in part to counter the darkness and shame that had surrounded cancer in the nineteenth century. The goals of bringing cancer experiences into public view and offering hope to people with cancer certainly provide productive outlets for responding to cancer. However, as is the case with war topoi, lines of argument urging a positive and even cheerful response to cancer ironically function to obscure the reality of the disease that is ostensibly being made visible. The hope that topoi of positivity might offer to cancer patients ultimately becomes secondary, as these topoi function primarily to create a people who can demonstrate moral and emotional strength in the face of all challenges, a feature of a eugenic mission to assert that the goals of social improvement can be pursued through the cultivation of the right attitude.

Arguments for hope and positivity, beginning in the 1930s and gaining scientific validation in the latter decades of the twentieth century, ultimately impose the burden of responsibility for controlling cancer on individuals who, in keeping with Roosevelt's "determined conquest" of polio, are imagined capable of conquering the disease through sheer force of will.[7] As Sara Ahmed points out, discourses of happiness often support not those who are tasked with demonstrating happiness but larger social systems that depend upon the reassurance that all is in order: "We learn from this history how happiness is used as a technology or instrument, which allows the reorientation of individual desire toward a common good."[8] The topoi of positivity therefore can be seen as examples of the euthenic discourse that Currell describes as a "self-improvement formula" infused with eugenic ideologies and serving the purpose of social advancement more than the interests of those it ostensibly benefits.[9]

CANCER AND DESPAIR

Even ancient views of cancer assumed a physiological connection between the disease and negative emotions. In *Emperor of All Maladies,* Siddhartha Mukherjee discusses the ancient Greek physician Galen's application of Hippocrates's theory that all diseases can be accounted for through studying the balance of bodily fluids. Galen believed that cancer, like melancholy, was the result of an excess of black bile, which linked cancer and depression. Galen considered cancer treatment futile, since tumors were caused by trapped bile, evidence of "a deep-seated bodily dysfunction" that could not be eradicated through surgery.[10] Mukherjee notes that this view influenced medicine for centuries following Galen's death in 199 AD, which helps to account for the shame associated with a disease that was for centuries "synonymous with filth and decay."[11] As discussed in chapter 1, this view was challenged in the twentieth century as the medical community rallied around the cause of eradicating the shame of cancer in order to promote early detection. At the same time, the challenge to the stigma surrounding cancer did not entirely eliminate the suspicion that dispositional causes might account for the presence of the disease, a view that surprisingly gained force over the decades of the twentieth century.

The vocabulary describing the nature of the "deep-seated bodily dysfunction" varied across centuries. James Olson references French physician Pierre Dionis's theory that "such psychic forces as sorrow and anger might cause a coagulation of lymphatic fluids in a woman's breast and produce a tumor"; the link between cancer and depression posited by New York physician William Parker in 1885; the argument of James Paget, a nineteenth-century British surgeon, that depression should be considered "a weighty additive to the other influences favoring the development of a cancerous constitution"; and the 1940s theory of Wilhelm Reich, an Austrian psychotherapist, that cancer is the result of a "chronic emotional calm" that reflected a deficiency of the "orgone energy" needed for sexual fulfillment and a satisfactory life.[12]

Although the Food and Drug Administration challenged Reich's orgone therapy in 1954,[13] these examples illustrate the resilience of ancient ideas linking cancer and depression. At the same time, improvements in cancer treatment meant that a cancer diagnosis was no longer an automatic death sentence, a fact that called for approaches to working with cancer patients that would emphasize possibilities for fulfilling lives after cancer. Thus, interest in the cancer patient's state of mind ranged from the practical goal of rescuing people with cancer from bleak hospital wards whose dark halls symbolized the hopelessness that had been attached to their fate in earlier eras to arguments concerning the beneficial effects of positivity on mental and physical health. While shifts in arguments for positivity respond to changing cultural contexts, the persistent presence of topoi pertaining to positivity and cheerfulness fuse ancient assumptions concerning the dispositional causes of cancer with eugenic goals to promote the improvement of the race through improving the physical and mental fitness of individuals.

CANCER, HOPE, AND THE WHOLE PATIENT

The persistent suspicion that cancer might be caused by despair and stress obviously has negative implications. At the same time, twentieth-century developments in cancer diagnosis and treatment also featured a more productive framework for attending to the psychological health of the patient and connecting cancer treatment to a hopeful outlook. In addition to simply making cancer a subject that could be talked about, the effort to promote public awareness drew upon the rhetorical function of space to create cancer treatment centers that made visible the hopeful message that twentieth-century cancer advocates wanted to share. This spirit is evident in a 1935 article about Memorial Hospital, titled "A Cheerful Institution," which links the positive atmosphere of the hospital to the change in public attitudes toward cancer, as well as the prognosis of patients who seek early treatment: "A visitor to the hospital finds it not a gloomy, but a cheerful place. A more wholesome public attitude toward cancer is reflected in the large number of persons who come to the clinics for early advice and prompt treatment when the chances of recovery are most favorable. There is also the cheerfulness of a staff devoted to its task of alleviating human suffering."[14] At times, the hospital combined its effort to brighten the environment with activities for patients. A 1939 *New York Herald Tribune* article titled "Getting Ready for Christmas" describes the role of hospitalized children in providing holiday decorations: "The shining glass partitions of one of the world's most unusual hospital wards began to take on a holiday dress of gay colors yesterday as four young patients set to work on the special decorations in their temporary home, the children's ward at the Memorial Hospital."[15] Such efforts to keep patients occupied during a difficult hospitalization certainly represent an improvement over earlier approaches that assumed that cancer patients should assume an attitude of grim resignation or even shame.

Advances in treatment by the middle of the century extended this optimistic view of the plight of the cancer patient. The goal of making cancer facilities bright and cheerful became increasingly prominent in the decades following the opening of the new Memorial Hospital; a September 25, 1951, press release documenting the opening of a new clinic dedicated by Eleanor Roosevelt states, "Throughout the new building the accent is on cheerfulness. Each floor is brightened by a special washable wall covering in a different gay design. Modern fluorescent lighting fixtures, white soundproof ceilings and sunlit examining rooms add to both the hopeful atmosphere and efficiency of the individual clinic areas."[16] These attractive surroundings were accompanied by a concerted effort on the part of major cancer centers to encourage patients to see their environment as a physical representation of their hope for a positive outcome.

Ongoing improvements in the prognosis of cancer patients in subsequent decades continued to be reflected in arguments for new medical representations of cancer. The 1964 announcement of a new facility by Memorial

Sloan Kettering Cancer Center president Richard D. Vanderwarker contains explicit discussion of the need for environments that reflect the changing landscape of cancer care, including practical implications pertaining to the increased longevity of people with cancer: "When Memorial Hospital was founded in 1884, it was concerned primarily with providing aid and comfort to the dying. Today the keynote of our institution is the cured cancer patient . . . This change in attitude and goal can be seen readily in our construction plans which will include a minimal care unit. More and more patients are being cured every year, and the minimal care unit not only makes the transition between hospital and home easier for the patient following treatment, but also will provide care at a more acceptable economic level."[17] As was the case with the topos of cancer as battle, the evolving topos of cheer persistently connected material conditions, developments in medical treatment, and the well-being of cancer patients and their families.

In addition to changing facilities, the increasingly hopeful outlook led to a new approach in training the medical staff that supported cancer patients, as well as diversifying the roles of individuals responsible for patient care. In a 1949 article in the *American Journal of Nursing* titled "Raising the Cancer Patient's Morale," Caroline Keller writes, "The problem of developing an understanding of the patient's personality-in-illness becomes particularly urgent in the treatment of patients who enter a hospital known to be solely devoted to the treatment of cancer."[18] Keller stresses the need for nurses to prepare themselves to maintain a hopeful attitude that can inspire patients to do the same. The press release summarizing the Memorial Hospital report delivered by board of managers president Laurance Rockefeller in December 1951 describes the improved prognosis of Memorial patients as partly due to a shift from a medical team focused only on the patient's survival to a broader network of support aimed at "care of the patient as a whole": "Because of these ever-increasing cure rates, the activities of Memorial, as described in the report, are being built around the restitution of the cancer patient as a productive, happy member of society. This has resulted in a larger more complicated team which now requires psychiatrist, psychologist, recreational therapist and administrator to function as actively and intimately with the patient as does the physician, surgeon, nurse and social worker."[19]

During the 1950s, Arthur M. Sutherland, a psychiatrist on the staff of Memorial Hospital, conducted extensive research that broke new ground in understanding and communicating about the total well-being of cancer patients. In his portrait of Sutherland's work, Michael Braun notes that Sutherland's attention to the psychological health of the cancer patient came about in an environment in which "technological considerations were paramount and psychosocial ones still under challenge as an avenue of legitimate inquiry."[20] Sutherland's 1954 speech to the Sixth International Cancer Congress in São Paulo, Brazil, warns of "psychological invalidism" that threatens the well-being of cancer patients and their families. Sutherland notes that "almost all cancer patients have difficulty in adjusting to the disease and the methods used in its cure," but argues for a close working relationship among families, physicians, and patients in order to help patients and families navigate the challenges of cancer care.[21]

Developments at Memorial Hospital in subsequent decades continued to emphasize the care of the whole patient. A 1960 address commemorating the seventy-fifth anniversary of Memorial's Nursing Division delivered by Sister Charles Marie Frank, dean of the School of Nursing of the Catholic University of America, eloquently calls for "the ideal 'American humanist' attitude reflected by the nurse who approaches the patient with full respect for his dignity, his rights, and his freedom."[22] Frank insists that competent treatment is no longer adequate, as those nurses "trained just to excel in technical efficiency" will not be equipped to treat patients with the compassion they deserve: "Sickness may strip a patient of his liberty but that does not justify us to strip him of his dignity. Our authority over him places additional responsibility upon us to maintain that dignity."[23] Frank insists that such an approach not only improves the experience of the cancer patient but also adds to the job satisfaction of medical professionals.

This view is echoed in the next decade in a public affairs press release dated October 26, 1977, announcing the creation of a research center for cancer nursing. Marilyn T. Oberst, the nursing research director, contrasts disease treatment and health care, adding, "An essentially biological view of illness, while appropriate for the science of cure, is inadequate for the study of health care because it doesn't account for the interaction between state of health and human behavior."[24] The following year, the hospital opened a psychiatry service described as "the first contemporary full-time psychiatric service in a cancer hospital in this country," providing training for "psychiatrists, residents and oncologists in the special needs of the cancer patient."[25] This focus yielded useful insight that held immediate benefits to cancer patients. In a May 14, 1979, speech to the American Society for Clinical Oncology, Dr. Mary Jane Massie, clinical assistant psychiatrist at Memorial, refers to depression as the most frequent cause for psychiatric consultation, adding, "Depression in cancer patients should not be regarded as an inevitable accompaniment of cancer."[26] Greater attention to varied ways of enhancing the full range of experiences surrounding treatment and its aftermath, including attention to the relationship between mental health and chronic disease, helps to account for the improved quality of life available to cancer patients in the latter decades of the twentieth century.

The notion that the optimal cancer treatment is carried out by teams of professionals was established in other cancer centers during the same period. The MD Anderson annual report from 1950–51 includes sections devoted to nursing, social service, volunteer services, and psychosomatic medicine. Staff members in each category are described as contributing to a team effort to support the full range of patients' needs. The report stresses the recognition that nurses "must be sensitive to the emotional and social problems related to the disease and work with the doctors, social worker, psychologist, etc. in an effort to achieve a reasonable adjustment," while the social service unit focused on three dimensions: "The Service to the Patient, The Service to the Hospital, The Service to the Community." With the assistance of professionals, the patient "is helped to adjust to the demands of treatment and accept the limitations of the disease; recognize the social situations that interfere with medical care and meet the many problems peculiar to his illness: financial, family, and personal."[27]

The report from that year also reveals how attention to fulfilling patient needs outside of the strict boundaries of physical health connected with various outreach efforts on MD Anderson's part. The hospital's Social Service Department established connections with "interested racial groups" who were encouraged to engage with the particular needs of cancer patients from marginalized communities. Unfortunately, during this period an accompanying feature of this initiative was the segregation of the hospital's services. The 1948 meetings with "Negro and Spanish leaders" ultimately led to the 1950 opening of a sixteen-bed facility called "the Negro Annex," with the anticipation of an equivalent facility guided by the efforts of "the Spanish group" in the future. The hospital's decision to employ Beatrix Cobb, at that time a research fellow completing her doctoral dissertation, was also discussed in the 1950–51 report. This initial report explicitly linked Cobb's hiring to the view that early detection efforts depended upon understanding the cancer patient's state of mind, emphasizing her contribution to "an effort toward a more comprehensive understanding of the underlying causes of delay in seeking medical assistance on the part of individuals with cancer." The report suggests that this initial study will yield greater insight into "the place of the clinical psychologist in a cancer hospital . . . and that a permanent place will be made available for a psychologist to be on the staff of the MD Anderson Hospital."[28]

The notion of cancer treatment as requiring a team of professionals equipped to address the mental, physical, and emotional needs of the patient continued to be emphasized in both the Memorial Sloan-Kettering and MD Anderson Cancer Centers in subsequent decades. An October 14, 1968, Memorial Sloan-Kettering press release emphasizes the importance of all staff members in supporting the well-being of the patient, including "researchers, clinicians, nurses, technicians, aides, volunteers, security men, dieticians, laundry workers, maintenance men, engineers and many others," adding, "It is an underlying principle of the institution that treating cancer is not enough. The patient must be comfortable and able to function as a productive member of society."[29] This approach assumed the worthy goal of promoting a positive atmosphere that would be sustained by all staff members associated with the care of cancer patients, a useful counter to the atmosphere of doom that often pervaded nineteenth-century cancer wards.

The emphasis on hope, support for the whole patient, and the maintenance of normal activities led to the promotion of social opportunities that would assure cancer patients that opportunities for fulfilling lives were available to them no matter how profound the physical consequences of the disease and its treatment. An April 1951 Memorial Hospital press release anticipates with enthusiasm the annual dinner dance of the Amputees Alliance, a group formed in 1948 by two surgeons from Memorial's Bone Tumor Service: "Ballroom dancing will be an important part of the evening's festivities. These amputees believe they can do whatever their two-legged friends can do and sometimes are spurred to do more."[30] The writer explains the organization's purpose as not only offering social fulfillment to those who have lost limbs but also assuring people diagnosed with bone cancer that their lives have not effectively ended with their diagnosis. The press release describes the organization's audience as including "the ill who required amputation and yet refused thinking death would be preferable to life minus an extremity."[31] The desire to offer a positive alternative to debilitating despair can be seen as a driving force in this social event, as well as many others organized by cancer centers during this era.

In addition to supporting dances for amputees, Memorial Hospital launched an annual patients' art exhibition in the late 1940s that was sustained for many years. A March 1966 press release announces the recreation department's sponsorship of the nineteenth annual Patients' Art Exhibition, adding:

> For most of the 50 artists who participate in the show each year, the classes they attended when they were patients were their first "brush," pun intentional, with art. For example, there is the 65-year-old business executive whose right arm was amputated three years ago and who learned to paint with his left hand.
>
> "Our art classes and shows have come to have a double meaning," says Mrs. Wilkinson. "They serve the initial purpose for which they were set up—constructive use of leisure time by the patient well enough to participate. But the extra dividend is hope. When a patient hears about others who have been in straits similar to his and who not only are well five to ten years later, but painting, you can imagine the boost it gives him."[32]

The fusion of hope with activity and entertainment is also increasingly evident across the MD Anderson annual reports from the 1950s. The 1951–52 annual report details the goals of the Medical Social Service department, which encompass "general patient welfare, case work services and community organization." The report explains that the department's philosophy is grounded in an emphasis on offering varied services "to the patient so that his interest and cooperation will be aroused." In response to this challenge, the report explains that the department has "developed handicraft programs, supplied entertainment including television shows, encouraged and conducted hobby displays, arranged friendly visiting groups, developed a community flower service, and effected a reading service, all to the end that the patient will be happier during his stay and course of treatment." The report also details support provided from the volunteer service, which included not only entertainment, but also rehabilitation programs designed to prepare patients for their return to community life. In addition to handicraft classes aimed at helping patients develop employable skills, volunteer groups took on special projects such as bucco-esophageal speech training class for patients whose treatment involved surgical removal of the larynx. Traditional entertainment was also emphasized, including daily volunteer visits, which included segregated volunteer groups who were seen as particularly well prepared to address "the special needs of the Negro patients," visiting talent presentations, and outings to participate in community activities. The 1951–52 report also boasts the benefits available through the opening of the new "home for Spanish-speaking patients which was made possible by the interest and efforts of a group of Houston citizens."[33] The development of programs to promote connections between cancer patients and the world beyond the hospital included measures that also brought constraints of the outside world, including racial segregation, into the hospital.

Throughout the 1950s, MD Anderson worked to expand the network of programs that distracted patients from the challenges surrounding their treatment, ensured their continued engagement with the external world in spite of those challenges, and prepared them for life beyond the immediate limitations that illness imposed upon them. The 1952–53 annual report boasts of the quality of the hospital's handicraft program, noting that "in several instances patients who previously have been unable to support themselves and their dependents have made a gainful occupation of one of the handicraft trades." Meanwhile, the expansion of the volunteer service facilitated a more ambitious program to engage patients with the community around them. The volunteer service report notes that "in addition to the activities conducted at the Annex, the patients are taken on weekly drives around the city, to the circus, ice shows, rodeos, horse shows and as many passive diversions as conform to the rules and regulations of the hospital." Although the report does not state that most of the benefits described are designed to serve white patients, it does provide a separate discussion of benefits available to African American patients: "During the current year, the Negro Gray Ladies have organized a similar recreation and entertainment group and have purchased a television set for the negro annex." In addition, plans continued for the care of Latinx patients through the purchase of La Posada, a home for Spanish-speaking outpatients. The report notes the ways in which such strategies are directly connected to the physical and emotional well-being of patients: "The awareness of the needs of the cancer patients by many individuals as well as the previously described groups have made it possible to relieve the anxieties of many by better understanding and individual care. Acceptance of long and difficult treatment has been easier because of the happiness and comfort provided during hospitalization."[34]

By 1954–55, MD Anderson had extended its range of services to include a beauty shop for patients. Special programs were also in place for the children's ward. In addition to "organized plays, holiday parties, Sunday School, television, professional story-tellers, artists, trips to the zoo," the ward enjoyed celebrity visits: "Visits by Annie Oakley, Gene Autry and others were a great treat. Particularly fine were autographed baseballs by the Indians, the Buffs, and the Cardinals (who also sent an autographed picture, in color of all members of the team and a Certificate of Membership in the Association of Honorary Bat Boys) sent to a 13-year-old lad who had been the star of his school baseball team until he lost his right leg to cancer; and an autographed football from Rice Institute's team which was presented by the coach and players to a youthful football player who also had lost a limb." The report continues to emphasize the intricate links between the positive environment supported by social service activities and the goal of removing the dread and fear of cancer that had in earlier eras inhibited early detection: "The Cancer Care Institutes, held for the first time in 1953 have become an annual project of medical social service. The institutes have been planned and carried out primarily as educational media for social workers, public health nurses and vocational rehabilitation counselors from all parts of the state who are in a strategic position to encourage cancer patients to seek medical care in the early stages of their disease."[35]

By the end of the 1950s, the annual reports highlight the role of volunteer services as parallel to that of medical professionals. While medical professionals focused their attention on the patient's physical needs, volunteers served the vital role of providing emotional support to patients and serving as a bridge to the community. The volunteer services section in the 1959–60 MD Anderson annual report states, "The purposes of this service are to release the professional from the nonprofessional aspects of his work and to create a volunteer program so satisfying to the workers that they will interpret the hospital functions and needs to the community."[36] This general idea is sustained in the decades that follow, and in the 1974–76 annual report is explicitly tied to the recognized material needs of patients who come from long distances to receive medical care at the hospital: "The primary function of the MD Anderson Hospital volunteer is to provide personal services and attention and thereby improve patient care and comfort. They also release professional and allied health personnel from nonprofessional duties. Many of the services they perform for the cancer patient and his family could not otherwise be provided and are especially important at MD Anderson Hospital, since most of the patients are away from their home communities."[37] At this point, the hospital's structure created something of a division between physical and emotional health, but there was a continued assumption that the medical community had some obligation to attend to every dimension of the patient's experience, an assumption that usefully countered the secrecy and debilitating fears of the past and that continues to be a feature of cancer centers in the present day.

CANCER, HOPE, AND CURE: THE DARK SIDE OF POSITIVITY

Documents from the latter decades of the twentieth century reflect increased attention on the part of both institutions to preparing patients for life after cancer. A 1978 speech by J. Herbert Dietz, chief of the Memorial Sloan-Kettering's Rehabilitation Service, quoted in a Memorial Sloan-Kettering News press release, describes the cancer center's emphasis on a team effort focused on "helping cancer patients to adapt and to return to their families and society."[38] Many of the benefits associated with efforts to encourage patients to pursue a full and active life are highlighted in a 1988 issue of MD Anderson's *Conquest* magazine, which features the stories of various advances that have made it possible for patients to resume the lives they led before cancer. This goal is explicitly discussed by speech pathologist Julia Bowman in an article titled "Functional Living Means Talking": "What we want for our patients is a return to the lives they led before their illnesses. . . . Hospital-based training and the patients' homework provide pathways for their return to functional lives after cancer."[39] Another article, "Matching Desire and Potential," extends Bowman's specific focus on helping those with cancer affecting the vocal cords to regain the ability to speak to other aspects of an active and fulfilling life. This article quotes Barbara Shell, MD Anderson's director of physical therapy, as stating that "'depending on their physical status and how fully they recuperate, cancer patients can aspire to about any activity they want—jogging, golf, returning to careers or just working around the house. . . . Although cancer causes physical changes for most patients, those changes don't have to limit the fullness of their lives."[40]

An underlying theme running through much of the discourse surrounding improvements in the emotional health of the cancer patient is the notion of control. While control over one's destiny can be seen as a desirable objective, problematic implications emerge from the frequent connections among control, cheerfulness, and positivity. Topoi urging a positive attitude toward cancer often shift seamlessly from the valuable focus on helping people with cancer pursue fulfilling lives to broader goals that entail rhetorically constituting a people committed to managing a disease represented as an unnecessary intrusion in a modern society's eugenic quest for perfection. The obsession with positivity therefore moves from the desirable goal of integrating cancer into ordinary life to a problematic emphasis on an idealized response to cancer that protects society at large from the need to confront the complicated and oftentimes negative reality of the disease. The lines of argument that emerge across the twentieth century are often based in modern psychological theories, but they reflect to a surprising degree ancient assumptions concerning the mysterious link between cancer and the humors. The papers of Frederick L. Hoffman, the Prudential Insurance Company statistician who provided data influential to the study of cancer during the early decades of the twentieth century, reflect varying views of cancer's relationship to the mind during that period. Hoffman's notes for a lecture titled "The Control of Cancer" feature a bulleted list of talking points that include "Cancer not infectious or contagious," "Cancer not caused by heredity," and "Cancer not caused by worry."[41] However, Hoffman's handwritten note attached to a 1916 *Scientific American* article by Cyrus Topliff titled "The Cancer Problem" describes the article as a summary of "all that is officially known about cancer, up to the present time"; according to the note, this knowledge includes attention to the relationship between the mind and body that suggests "if fear, worry, hate, spite, jealousy, and all irritating thoughts, were entirely eliminated from the mind, then cancer, and all inflammatory forms of disease, would probably not develop in the body; and cases where the disease is already present, if not too far advanced could, no doubt, be cured."[42] The notion that disease might be eradicated through somehow ensuring that "all irritating thoughts, were entirely eliminated from the mind" resonates with *Physical Culture*'s euthenic philosophy of "increasing human efficiency and health by improving the way humans interacted with and controlled their environment."[43]

The subtle lines between the desire to support the whole person and the move to attribute disease to mental or emotional deficiency are consistently blurred in twentieth-century cancer topoi. Curtis E. Lakeman's 1915 assurance that individuals can manage their cancer through "strength of mind and will" offers reassurance that a cancer diagnosis does not mean that all is lost.[44] However, it also implicitly supports the eugenic view that people with access to certain social, mental, physical, and emotional resources are destined to thrive, while those who do not fare well may not have had the qualities needed to overcome the disease. Such arguments not only signal the individual's capacity to determine the outcome of cancer treatment but also construct a people convinced that all obstacles to achieving the norm, including strength, health, and an able body, can be eliminated through an appropriate disposition. A section in a 1988 *Conquest* issue titled "Getting on with Life" emphasizes this goal in discussing advances in pain control. Dr. C. Stratton Hill, MD Anderson's director of pain service, states, "What we most need to do is improve the way we manage cancer patients' pain so they have a sense of being in charge."[45]

Of course, the emphasis on alleviating the suffering of cancer patients is unequivocally positive, as are stories that capture the resiliency of individuals who have resisted the limitations cancer might have imposed on them through determination and positivity, as well as support from others. An article in the same *Conquest* issue titled "A Nurse's Brag Book" tells the story of an enterostomal therapist who helps patients adjust to rerouting procedures of bladder and bowels. The article features a patient who refused to abandon his active life following a urinary ostomy: "Strack's determination was obvious as he practiced wearing the bags before surgery and in the way he managed the new method of voiding after the operation last April. Still an avid outdoorsman at fifty-one, Strack vowed to be back water skiing by mid-summer." The story goes on to describe Strack's "mechanical ingenuity" in adjusting the physical constraints involved in his medical condition so that he could wear jeans, minimize bathroom breaks while traveling in his pickup, and sleep through the night. In addition, Strack credits the support of his wife, who continued to run their business during the most intense period of his illness and "also drove the boat and pulled him on a slalom ski exactly three months after his surgery." Strack's story is indeed remarkable, and it is certainly appropriate to celebrate with him as he concludes, "Making these modifications gives me a sense of control."[46]

At the same time, it is difficult to escape the question of who benefits most from stories highlighting the possibility of control and the benefits of a positive response to cancer. An early mascot for cancer positivity was Dorothy Lewis, an eight-year-old whose treatment for bone cancer received substantial media attention in 1939. The widespread news coverage of Lewis, whose cancer also required the amputation of a leg, illustrates the public's craving for cheerful stories about cancer. A *New York Journal American* story juxtaposes Lewis's tearful response to a toothache with her cheerful outlook on cancer: "Dorothy, who amazed the medical world with her courage and her recuperative powers after surgeons severed her leg, was soon smiling again after a sedative had been administered to relieve the pain of an aching back molar."[47] The section of the article titled "Great Progress" assures the reader that the removal of the offending tooth enabled Dorothy to regain her typical cheerfulness: "With all the resourcefulness of youth, the brave little cancer victim was making great progress—even having fun—getting about on her new crutches. Her blue eyes sparkled as she hopped about to display her prowess to a visitor."[48] Other newspapers carried stories highlighting Lewis's cheerful response, such as the photo caption published in the *Shenandoah Herald* (Shenandoah, Pennsylvania) that refers to Lewis's smile as a "bright badge of courage."[49] These stories offer the array of emotions described by Rosemarie Garland-Thomson, as the reader is allowed to move from "pity, fear, discomfort, guilt" to the "sense of normalcy" that comes from the assurance that Lewis's illness has not prevented her from having fun on her crutches.[50]

Dorothy Lewis's plight invokes the audience's awareness about the threat of cancer, but her "bright badge of courage" helps to make the emotion more bearable through assuring readers that it is possible to handle the horror of the disease. The stigma associated with disease and disability therefore becomes manageable not through awareness that leads to social change but through the attitude of those whose health places them outside the mainstream: "The stigmatized individual is asked to act so as to imply neither that his burden is heavy nor that bearing it has made him different from us . . . So deeply, then, must he be caught up in the attitude to the self that is defined as normal in our society, so thoroughly must he be a part of this definition, that he can perform this self in a faultless manner to an edgy audience that is half-watching him in terms of another show."[51] Thus, the heightened visibility of Dorothy Lewis's cheerfulness subtly shifts attention from the complex range of experiences she faces and creates a people confident that even the most debilitating effects of cancer can be overcome by those who maintain the right outlook.

The public's confidence in the potential to control cancer through the right disposition often leads to unrealistic expectations. Olson argues that the cancer experience of athlete Mildred "Babe" Didrikson Zaharias in the early 1950s was in part responsible for a turn to "the modern culture of an unrealistic assumption: that optimism and willpower could cure cancer."[52] Although Zaharias died three years after her diagnosis, Olson describes her frankness and positive outlook as having done "much to mitigate the stigma of colon cancer and render it just a disease, not a metaphor for filth and disgust."[53] Eliminating the attitude of disgust toward cancer is certainly a productive outcome, but the circulation of arguments focused on strength and positivity often results in cyclical claims about the power of individuals to determine the course of their disease, while those who have not had good outcomes are implicitly assumed as somehow failing to cultivate the qualities needed to improve their prognosis. These arguments ultimately shift the audience's attention from the uncertainty surrounding any cancer diagnosis to an idealized representation of the sick person whose capacity to "look on the bright side" functions primarily as "a lesson for the nondisabled."[54] As S. Lochlann Jain points out, the pressure to conceal the ravages of cancer subordinates the needs of those dealing with the disease to larger public interests: "We know cancer will happen, yet when it does, it seems dishonoring or indecorous. I don't refer to its side-effects here;

the physical breakdown of the body virtually epitomizes 'indecorousness.' Judgments about proper decorum (*be a survivor, wear a wig, look good!*) can help illuminate the ugly downside of America's will to health."[55]

THE IMPERATIVE OF POSITIVITY

Certainly there is much to be said for a positive outlook in providing strength to people who encounter difficult situations. However, the blurring of the lines between hope and blame repeatedly begs the question of who is actually being addressed by topoi of positivity. Ehrenreich's insistence that the concerted emphasis on positive thinking imposes pressure on patients that does more harm than good is certainly a negative potential outcome of these arguments. But the primary goal of topoi of positivity is neither to bolster the spirits of people with cancer nor to blame them for their plight; rather, it is to create a people confident that they live in a society in which beneficial outcomes are available to those with the right physical and dispositional qualities. The goal of offering productive outlets for countering the helplessness that often accompanies a cancer diagnosis is an important one, but the imposition of a positive outlook serves social aims that are connected with eugenic goals that function independently of the circumstances of individuals.

As is the case with the topos of cancer as war, the public insistence on cheer subordinates the needs of cancer patients to a cultural thirst for assurance that social progress is still achievable in spite of evidence that an incapacitating illness may strike anyone at any time. This is where the urgency for blame can be located, as a people determined to assert the perfectability of society must ensure that those whose health or ability places them outside the accepted norm are engaged in the process by which the "deficient adjustment is declared normalizable."[56] And many people with cancer are eager to assure themselves and others that they illustrate the desirable behaviors that enable them to maintain their membership in "the realm of the normal" despite their disease.[57] In a 1960 CBS reports interview titled "Biography of a Cancer," Dr. Dooley, a cancer patient from Laos recently diagnosed with melanoma, shares with reporter Howard K. Smith his goal of embodying a positive outlook that can offer a sense of hope to people who have been diagnosed with cancer: "There's a certain amount of ignorance in America about this word 'cancer.' The very minute they hear the word 'cancer,' Americans picture gloom, doom, and death. This makes people crippled before they even get crippled. That makes them mentally crippled when they come to the hospital." While Dooley acknowledges the problem caused by excessive fear and ignorance about cancer and effectively presents his own case as evidence that people "need not be so fearful of cancer," his subsequent reflections focus critical attention on the problem caused by specific individuals who are not able to maintain his outlook. One example is a woman whose response to her diagnosis with "a very insignificant type of cancer" involved a level of despair that he found unproductive: "She was a headache because she was ignorant. She was ignorant because perhaps she hadn't seen a TV show that explains a little bit better what cancer and cancer research is doing."[58] It is impossible to know whether Dooley is accurate in saying that the woman's level of anxiety was higher than her particular diagnosis warranted, and it may be possible that she would have benefited from information about her hopeful prognosis. The point, however, is not whether the woman's anxiety was appropriate but to question what would lead someone to engage in judgment of other people's attitudes and to characterize them as "a headache" and "ignorant." The rapid shift from reassurance to negative perceptions of patients whose response is deemed undesirable can be seen as a persistent feature of the cancer topos of cheer, illustrating Ehrenreich's claim that "positive thinking seems to be mandatory in the breast cancer world, to the point that unhappiness requires a kind of apology."[59] The assumption that those who cannot emulate the "normal" characteristics identified by Stiker, "white, male, young, healthy, handsome, educated, and . . . submissive!," are somehow blameworthy is also part of the ongoing legacy of eugenic ideologies.[60] The woman in Dr. Dooley's example may not have been a problem because she had cancer, but she became a "headache" because her "ignorance" did not allow her to manage her illness with the positive spirit that would reassure others that the norm can be sustained even in light of a diagnosis that might suggest the contrary. Thus, intelligence, education, and stoic strength of will become the qualities that can overcome the problem of cancer.

CHEERFULNESS AND HEALTH

In addition to suggesting that the cancer patient's inability to maintain a positive attitude might be seen as a character flaw, Ehrenreich notes another source of pressure: the view that "a 'positive attitude' is somehow essential to recovery."[61] And in fact the early twentieth-century views that cancer might be eliminated "if fear, worry, hate, spite, jealousy, and all irritating thoughts, were entirely eliminated from the mind," that cancer "is purely a question of the individual and his strength of mind," are fully developed in later theories that draw more explicit connections among mental and emotional health and the prognosis of the cancer patient.[62] In "Think About It: The Misbegotten Promise of Positive Thinking Discourse," Louise Woodstock outlines a long history of positive thinking defined by the premise that "unhappiness and disease are social fabrications and that society, in turn, infects individuals with misconceptions about reality."[63] The notion that physical and social disease are linked squarely aligns cancer rhetorics of positivity with the eugenic impulse to cure society through addressing individual deficiencies. Woodstock describes mind-cure pioneer Phineas Quimby's view that "disease was a social fabrication" as a foundation for the corollary belief that "an individual's body, as physical material, was also constructed by the individual's thoughts."[64] Woodstock traces such lines of argument from the late nineteenth century into the middle decades of the twentieth, as they reappear in Norman Vincent Peale's *The Power of Positive Thinking*, published in 1952, which suggests "a direct correlation between positive thoughts and positive consequences and, conversely, between negative thoughts and negative consequences."[65] As discussed in the previous chapter, the notion that the mind has at least partial control over physical health is also connected with the euthenic vision of Bernarr Macfadden, a vision driven by "intensified fears of further eugenic decay."[66]

The circulation of these ideas moved into the realm of cancer as a number of psychotherapists explored the notion of a "cancer personality" that accounted for weakened immune systems that caused cancer. The emergence of modern psychotherapy and attention to the workings of the unconscious provided a scientific lens for exploring the links between psychological and physical health. In response to an interview question about whether cancer might be a psychosomatic illness, Carl Jung states, "Well, you see, I couldn't swear, but I have seen cases where I thought or wondered whether or not there was a psychogenic reason for that particular ailment. . . . Many things can be found out about cancer, I'm sure. You see, with us it has been always a question of how to treat these things, because any disease possible has a psychological accompaniment. It just all depends upon—perhaps life depends upon it—whether you treat such a patient psychologically in the proper way or not. That can help tremendously, even if you cannot prove in the least that the disease in itself is psychogenic."[67] Jung's notion that "any disease possible has a psychological accompaniment" further developed a framework for advancing potential links between the body and the mental attitude of the patient, a line of inquiry that informed the development of positive psychology around the middle of the century.[68] Olson describes the widespread assumption during that period that "sexually repressed, emotionally contained cancer victims were responsible for their own illnesses."[69] The appointment of Beatrix Cobb to MD Anderson's medical psychology staff in 1951 points to the integration of this perspective into the work of major cancer centers at certain points in time; Olson describes Cobb's view as grounded in the supposition "that cancer patients suffered a variety of emotional maladies, including a 'loss of self-respect,' 'self-pity,' 'fear of death,' and anxiety disorders."[70] Although controversy surrounding Cobb's theories in part led R. Lee Clark Jr., head of MD Anderson, to eliminate the hospital's psychiatry and psychology divisions in 1958, her theories fuse ancient ideas concerning the connection between cancer and the humors with euthenic principles popular earlier in the century, a legacy that survived in varied social and medical contexts long after Cobb's departure from MD Anderson.

Arguments centering positive thinking in cancer treatment acquired further scientific force in the 1970s through the work of influential figures in psychotherapy such as Lawrence LeShan and O. Carl Simonton. Drawing from his work with terminally ill cancer patients, LeShan's 1977 *You Can Fight For Your Life: Emotional Factors in the Treatment of Cancer* cites Galen's ancient theory that cancer was caused by "a melancholy disposition" to support a claim that he makes "with great certainty: the presence of cancer is usually an indication that there is something else wrong in the life of the patient."[71] Although LeShan acknowledges the difficulty of making certain claims about the relationship between mind, body, and emotions, he nevertheless offers logically structured and authoritative arguments to advance radical conclusions about the link between cancer and the mind. His book describes the methodical steps he has taken to acquire quantitative as well as qualitative data that prove his claims, including his own psychological testing, information acquired from a large control group managed by an outside agency, and a series of case studies.[72] LeShan's conclusions center upon varied patterns that in his view account for the personality traits most susceptible to cancer: low self-esteem, the inability to advocate for oneself, and a sense of despair.[73] LeShan asserts with confidence that his ability to identify the "link between personality and cancer" could ultimately lead to "the possibility of reducing the risk of cancer for countless human beings."[74] He insists that through honest therapeutic sessions, he is able to help patients acquire the will to live, an outlook he contrasts with that of desiring life only because of a fear of death.[75]

Similar lines of thought are present in Simonton's 1978 publication *Getting Well Again: A Step-by-Step, Self-Help Guide to Overcoming Cancer for Patients and Their Families,* coauthored with Stephanie Matthews-Simonton and James Creighton, which strongly emphasizes the individual's responsibility for health: "Everyone participates in his or her health or illness at all times."[76] While the importance of the individual's relationship to health may be clear, Simonton and his colleagues go on to build a complex argument about the relationship between attitude and disease that veers into more controversial territory. After posing the question, "Why do some patients recover their health and others die, when the diagnosis is the same for both?" the book examines the phenomenon of patients whose recovery seems to be related to "the belief that they *exerted some influence over the course of their disease.*"[77] The task Simonton and his collaborators take upon themselves is summed up in a question: "If the difference between the patient who regains his health and the one who does not is in part a matter of attitude toward the disease and belief that he could somehow influence it, then, we wondered, how could we influence patients' belief in that positive direction?"[78] Simonton's "whole-person approach to cancer treatment" focuses on recapturing the "full human identity" that for many patients has been subsumed by a "cancer identity."[79] This effort to bring positive thinking into scientific discourses about cancer converged with long-standing notions of cancer's connection to despair, suspicions that cancer's cause might be connected with stress, assumptions that the "strength of mind" of cancer patients plays a role in their prognosis, and the eugenic assumption that weakness, debilitating illness, and disability can be overcome by those equipped to respond appropriately.

Simonton's representation of his theory enacts a delicate balance between bold claims about the healing potential of a positive attitude and accepted medical practices pertaining to cancer treatment. Although he firmly denies any intention of questioning the need for physical treatment, his argument for greater acceptance of "the psychosomatic connection with cancer" introduces lines of reasoning that shift the focus of cancer treatment from the body to the mind, which sustains ancient views of the link between cancer and disposition and also anticipates an emphasis on mounting a positive response to cancer that continues in the present day.[80] Simonton's conviction "that emotional and mental states play a significant role both in *susceptibility* to disease, including cancer, and in *recovery* from all disease" is manifested in an elaborate scale that measures stress factors alongside the occurrence of disease.[81] After citing numerous researchers whose studies aim at determining the psychological profile of cancer patients, he writes, "In addition to the studies cited, experience with our patients leaves no reasonable doubt in our minds of a link between certain emotional states and cancer."[82]

Simonton frames the notion of psychological susceptibility to cancer as good news, since he believes that his program offers help in countering the dispositional characteristics that might cause people to be vulnerable to the ravages of cancer. He describes susceptibility as based not simply in stress, but in "the way of reacting to stress," which means that his program, which includes an elaborate combination of relaxation, meditation, and visualization therapies, can be useful in countering the negative effects that might inhibit a patient's response to treatment.[83] Although Simonton never promises that his program guarantees the success of cancer treatment, he cites a study that finds "that a *positive attitude toward treatment was a better predictor of response to treatment than was the severity of the disease*" (emphasis in the original).[84] At the very least, Simonton assures his patients and their families that his approach will result in the state of being "*weller than well*," manifested in "psychological strength, a positive self-concept, a sense of control over their lives that clearly represent an improved level of psychological development."[85] As is the case with the war metaphor, the topos of positivity in cancer rhetoric achieves its power in part through the promise of control. In parallel with the "euthenics" orientation of *Physical Culture* magazine, Simonton applies to a cancer context the goal of "increasing human efficiency and health by improving the way humans interacted with and controlled their environment."[86] His conclusions resonate hauntingly with Macfadden's motto: "Sickness is a sin; don't be a sinner. Weakness is a crime; don't be a criminal."[87]

Simonton's discipline of stress management and control is carried forward in the work of Bernie S. Siegel, a surgeon whose 1986 *Love, Medicine, and Miracles* begins with an account of the professional transformation that occurred in 1978 when he attended Simonton's "Psychological Factors, Stress, and Cancer" workshop.[88] Siegel shared Simonton's interest in the psychological factors that shape the individual's susceptibility to cancer as well as Simonton's view that the medical community is unwilling to acknowledge the role of psychosomatic factors in cancer: "One problem with cancer statistics is that most self-induced cures don't get into the medical literature."[89] Like LeShan and Simonton, Siegel conceives the response to stress as the central factor that must be addressed: "Not everyone who suffers a tragic loss or stressful change in lifestyle develops an illness. The deciding factor seems to be how one copes with the problem."[90] Siegel cites a study indicating that "depressed men are twice as likely to get cancer as nondepressives," an outcome that supports his contention that depression involves "quitting or giving up," an attitude that leaves the patient highly vulnerable to the force of an aggressive disease such as cancer.[91]

Siegel's willingness to probe into the psychic causes of cancer is infused with eugenic hopes for overcoming disease through social improvement and the cultivation of "fitter families." His attention to "personality programming" begins with a comment on his own good fortune in having a loving family whose support, in his view, "conditioned me to be a survivor," in contrast with others whose upbringing might lead them to believe that "disease can be their way of finally satisfying their parents' wishes—or God's."[92] Siegel's emphasis on how the fitness of his family prepared him for physical and mental health has a striking lineage with positive eugenics, and he carries this idea forward in positing that an inferior upbringing generates passive personalities that lack the toughness needed to mount a vigorous response to cancer. Siegel notes that problematic home environments force individuals to search for love, ultimately generating the personality of the "compulsive giver," a type that he perceives to be particularly prominent among cancer patients whose tendency to "put the needs of others ahead of their own" makes them vulnerable, a theory that in some respects circles back to LeShan's view that a lack of assertiveness contributes to one's susceptibility to cancer. In fact, Siegel argues that "cancer might be called the disease of nice people," as it preys upon those who lack the strength of will to make their own goals central to their lives.[93]

While Siegel's course of treatment mirrors the emphasis on relaxation and meditation that Simonton outlines, he moves beyond his mentor in his confident assertions about his ability to make predictions about the relationship between physical health and mental outlook. While Siegel's stated goal of encouraging people to "raise a generation of children programmed to be loving and healthy" seems admirable on the surface, more troubling dimensions emerge in Siegel's design of a program for identifying "exceptional patients" as distinct from "ordinary ones."[94] This approach at times entails bold measures, such as Siegel's decision to interrupt his partner's consultation with a patient to offer his own assessment of the patient's mental state, summed up in the statement, "I don't think you really want to live."[95] Although Siegel admits that his conduct enraged the patient's wife, he insists that his confrontational technique led to a breakthrough in which the patient recognized that his defeatist attitude, based in his emotional response to his father's dementia, had in fact made him more inclined to give up on life after his cancer diagnosis. Siegel's assessment of the success of such tactics reinforces his insistence upon the value of psychological measures in achieving an accurate prognosis.

Siegel's bold confidence in intuitive measures to ascertain the physical condition of cancer patients extends to others who have received the benefits of his training. He explains that "the receptionist in my office is a pretty good diagnostician, basing her suppositions merely upon her contact with the new patient."[96] Apparently the ability to recognize the qualities that make a patient "exceptional" is not limited to those with formal medical training, nor does it require extensive time and contact. One can only imagine what superficial qualities Siegel and his receptionist identified as those that would signal a disinclination to live. Siegel's practices enact the eugenic framework of "sciences of the surface," which Snyder and Mitchell explain was a staple of nineteenth-century immigration and disability diagnosis: "Unlike their French counterparts, U.S. investigators of idiocy placed great emphasis on surface physical qualities as the route to an enlightened knowledge of 'peculiar mental conditions.' The body is transformed into a yet-to-be-explored topography, whose inner secrets will be revealed. . . . Correlations between physical and cognitive anomalies underwrite the legitimacy of 'sciences of the surface' and also offer an empirical method for differentiating among various categories of human beings—particularly those in need of moral and bodily uplift."[97] While Siegel was not focused on the discovery of idiocy, his claims that he and his staff were able to discern at a glance the physical and emotional qualities pointing toward an individual's fortitude in withstanding cancer demonstrate how the topos of positivity was infused with longstanding practices of superficial categorization associated with disability, an approach that Snyder and Mitchell describe as "the first stirrings of eugenic philosophy in the United States."[98]

The work of LeShan, Simonton, and Siegel is but a small sampling of the widespread interest in the relationship between positivity and cancer that entered mainstream cancer rhetoric during the 1970s and 1980s. And these lines of thought achieved such power because of the public's desire to believe them. In *Worried Sick: Our Troubled Quest for Wellness*, published two years after Siegel's book, Arthur J. Barsky notes that "the yearning to find psychological explanations for physical diseases runs deep," a phenomenon that is particularly pronounced in the search for connections between mental outlook and cancer survival.[99] Barsky references a controversial 1985 *New England Journal of Medicine* article "showing that psychological attitudes did *not* affect the progression of advanced cancers"; he adds that the article's conclusion that "more cheerful patients had no greater success than depressed ones in fighting their cancers" provoked a strongly negative public response.[100] He quotes the journal editor's recognition that the anger sparked by the article reflects the public's desire "to believe that how we think matters for our health—that we have the power to control things that are powerful and frightening."[101]

There are strains of good intention in many twentieth-century impulses to offer discourses of hope for cancer patients. Some aspects of the topos of positivity hold benefits similar to those that Martin E. P. Seligman and Mihaly Csikszentmihalyi identify within the field of positive psychology, which include helping people cultivate those strengths that will help them pursue fulfilling lives: "The field of positive psychology at the subjective level is about valued subjective experiences: well-being, contentment, and satisfaction (in the past); hope and optimism (for the future); and flow and happiness (in the present). At the individual level, it is about positive individual traits: the capacity for love and vocation, courage, interpersonal skill, aesthetic sensibility, perseverance, forgiveness, originality, future mindedness, spirituality, high talent, and wisdom. At the group level, it is about the civic virtues and the institutions that move individuals toward better citizenship: responsibility, nurturance, altruism, civility, moderation, tolerance, and work ethic."[102] This view recognizes that a positive frame of mind promotes strengths that potentially counter both mental and physical illness. The authors write, "The results of numerous studies of patients with life-threatening diseases, such as AIDS, suggest that those who remain optimistic show symptoms later and survive longer than patients who confront reality more objectively. . . . An optimistic patient is more likely to practice habits that enhance health and to enlist social support."[103]

While this way of describing the link between physical and emotional health seems reasonable, such lines of thought often move on to consider the possibility "that positive affective states may have a direct physiological effect that retards the course of illness."[104] The hazards of this view are obvious. As Barsky argues, "If we credit courage and optimism for cure and survival, then we may also be implying fault when the outcome is less happy. If we can make ourselves healthy with positive thinking, then poor health must result from negative thoughts, or a failure to express repressed feelings or become more assertive. . . . If this is so, the patient whose disease progresses or spreads may feel guilty as well as ill."[105] This engages patients in a difficult cycle, as the sense of guilt people feel when their disease is unresponsive is then considered to be further evidence of the personality that caused the problem in the first place. Although LeShan acknowledges that everyone may feel discouraged at times, he insists that "the cancer-prone personality . . . *always* has that feeling; it is a fundamental aspect of his total approach to life."[106] The widespread belief in the existence of a "cancer-prone personality" creates added pressure for people already burdened by urgings to assert control over their health, or at the very least to perform positivity that may not reflect the reality of what they are feeling, "approximating the signs of being happy—passing as happy—in order to keep things in the right place."[107]

The tension between the pressure to be happy and the complex emotions surrounding human experiences with illness creates a new burden for many people with cancer. In an article titled "The Tyranny of the Positive Attitude in America: Observation and Speculation," Barbara S. Held asks, "If there indeed now exists unprecedented pressure to accentuate the positive, could it then be that the pressure itself to be happy and optimistic contributes to at least some forms of unhappiness?"[108] The fact that Held poses the question about general states of mind and not specifically about cancer is telling; if pressure to be positive can create emotional challenges for the average person, how much more might this be the case for someone dealing with cancer?

Yet, as this chapter has shown, it is the person with cancer who has become particularly vulnerable to "the tyranny of positivity." Erving Goffman's discussion of the social world as a site in which individuals perform adherence to cultural norms illustrates this point: "As human beings we are presumably creatures of variable impulse with moods and energies that change from one moment to the next. As characters put on for an audience, however, we must not be subject to ups and downs."[109] C. McGrath, C. F. C. Jordens, K. Montgomery, and I. H. Kerridge describe positive thinking as "both a cultural expectation and a moral norm for cancer patients."[110] Barrie R. Cassileth argues that the emphasis on positivity emerged as a response to cultural conditions, as is the case with other examples of unorthodox cancer treatments. Cassileth identifies several major cultural beliefs that contribute to this trend. The first is the belief in personal autonomy, which is connected to a desire for control: "Cancer symbolizes the uncertainties and limitations of modern medicine. . . . It is our commonly held position that, as one writer stated unequivocally, 'the mind has the power to heal.' We do not say that about tuberculosis or syphilis or any disease that can be treated and cured. We do not say that where we have the comfortable sense of comprehension and control now missing to a large degree in cancer medicine."[111] Cassileth notes that the trend to positivity reflects a significant shift from earlier eras, when "we retreated in fear from this disease."[112] The shift in cancer topoi to an aggressively optimistic stance, described by Cassileth as "a typically American approach later symbolized by the phrase 'the war on cancer,'" reflects an ongoing pattern in which cancer rhetoric responds to the values, assumptions, and anxieties of the surrounding culture.[113] In addition, it demonstrates the persistence of a eugenic hope for the cultivation of attitudes and behaviors that can ensure national health and strength even in the face of evident challenges.

CANCER, POSITIVITY, AND EUGENICS

The early decades of the twentieth century saw a shift from a cancer rhetoric based in silence to topoi focused on bringing cancer into the public view. The aggressive stance of the war metaphor maintained a presence in cancer rhetoric throughout the century, but the topos of positivity offered a line of argument that might appear to be a welcome alternative to this militaristic response. Certainly, the emphasis on rehabilitation, hope, and measures to support cancer patients are productive ways of approaching cancer treatment. The medical community's recognition that effective responses to cancer must consider the physical and emotional toll of the disease led to a more comprehensive approach to cancer treatment, as well as bringing attention to the diverse needs of the individuals receiving that treatment. Dietz's 1978 speech reflects an important acknowledgment on the part of medical professionals that "patients have different needs and provide different responses. Age, type of cancer and disability, personality characteristics and emotional outlook are factors that have to be considered on an individual basis."[114] At the same time, this chapter has demonstrated ways in which the modern focus on the personality of cancer patients at certain points merges with eugenic measures that assign the responsibility for treatment outcomes to the bodies, minds, and wills of patients. The subtle connections between personality, hope, and cancer treatment generate topoi that gradually shift from positivity aimed at fostering hope and rehabilitation to the pursuit of control over the uncontrollable—and arguments that support the view that the strength of the race can come about through "fit families" who will equip children to withstand all challenges, including cancer.

The suggestion that control is possible to those who are determined enough, positive enough, or sufficiently committed to life ultimately imposes tremendous pressure on people who have cancer. In "Wish Me Well," a 1989 article published in *Ms.* magazine, Ruth Shereff describes her struggle with "the mind-cancer connection" following her diagnosis with advanced ovarian cancer at the age of forty-four.[115] Shereff squarely addresses the "pervasive" view that patients are responsible for cancer: "The mind-cancer connection—that is, you cause it, so you can cure it—is everywhere: on talk shows, in magazines, and on the best-seller list, where *Love, Medicine, and Miracles* by surgeon Bernie Siegel has had a two-year run."[116] Shereff is keenly aware of the self-doubt prompted by theories such as Siegel's, particularly since she received three copies of his book from well-meaning friends and relatives: "How could a doctor, a surgeon no less, be so smug and so disdainful of science? At the same time, I was terrified. What if he was right?"[117] As Cassileth notes, to portray a positive outcome as available to those who are heroic enough almost inevitably circulates "an implied message about those who fail to survive."[118] The focus on individual accountability subordinates the complexity that surrounds any lived encounter with cancer to the goal of social control: "Never mind that poverty, race, and occupation play a huge role in determining one's health status, the doctrine of individual responsibility means that the less-than-fit person is a suitable source not only of revulsion but resentment."[119] Azra Raza argues that the pressure to focus on the positive also affects medical professionals, who are expected to ignore the lived experiences of their patients in order to maintain the focus the public demands: "*Stay positive* is the refrain, as if it were a sin to voice the intense pain and suffering of cancer patients. Why are we so afraid to tell the stories of the majority who die? Why keep promoting the positive anecdote?"[120]

While critiques of positivity and blame are accurate and important, there is value in situating these concerns within a broader historical trajectory, which illuminates how cancer topoi of positivity resonate with eugenic discourses from preceding decades. Siegel's notion that people who demonstrate a particular form of assertiveness might be less prone to develop cancer, and his repeated boasts about the ability he and his staff possess to identify "exceptional" patients at a glance, has uncomfortable connections to degeneracy theory as well as to the eugenic assumption that those who possess superior powers are capable of determining weakness based on "sciences of the surface," a superficial aesthetic assessment that is almost certainly bound to biases that include race, class, ethnicity, and gender.[121] The suggestion that those who die may simply be those who didn't want to live in the first place reflects troubling ways in which common lines of argument in cancer rhetoric support the construction of a people committed to a eugenically inflected vision of public health as something earned by those with the right heredity, disposition, and access. As the next chapter will show, similar tension can be seen in arguments that ostensibly empower people through educating them about behaviors and measures that will prevent cancer but ultimately serve the purpose of fostering a people equipped to control their fear through locating vulnerability in the bodies of those who lack the "exceptional" commitment to health and material resources, including education and access to health care, that will sustain society's progress.[122]

The urge to press others toward happiness has deep cultural roots, based in part on the fact that "bodies marked as deviant provide an opportunity to solidify other social actors' beliefs in their own moral goodness and proximity to normative ideals."[123] A new orientation is required in order to challenge the longstanding impulse to expect others to support normative ideals through demonstrating their ability "to look on the bright side." Sara Ahmed describes such an orientation as follows:

> We might need to attend to bad feelings not in order to overcome them but *to learn by how we are affected by what comes near*, which means achieving a different relationship to all our wanted and unwanted feelings as an ethical resource. I think what is underestimated by affirmative ethics is the *difficulty* of giving our attention to—and sustaining our attention on—certain forms of suffering. The desire to move beyond suffering in reconciliation, the very will to "be over it" by asking others to "get over it," means that those who persist in their unhappiness become causes of the unhappiness of many. Their suffering becomes transformed into our collective disappointment that we cannot simply put such histories behind us. Ethics cannot be about moving beyond pain toward happiness or joy without imposing new forms of suffering on those who do not or cannot move in this way.[124]

The power and reach of arguments for positivity in the face of adversity will make such an ethical vision difficult to pursue, but a first step lies in recognizing the eugenic resonances that permeate the demand that people with cancer demonstrate their fitness, seize control of their fate, and cultivate the cheerful response that others hope to see in them. While there is a place for hope in the cancer experience, to impose on others the goal of getting over the pain will ultimately lead to "new forms of suffering on those who do not or cannot move in this way."[125]

4

Knowledge, Power, and Cancer Prevention

After reviewing the family history outlined in my chart, my primary care physician urged me to consider genetic cancer screening. I explained my reasons for being uncertain about the value of the testing, but he responded with a battery of arguments aimed at persuading me otherwise: "I did the testing not for myself, but for my children," after which he added, "Knowledge is power!" Although I persevered in declining the test, I left the appointment with the vague sense that I had done a disservice to my family along with rejecting an opportunity to acquire knowledge that might enable me to control my destiny.

The lines of argument my doctor used are broadly consistent with the cancer topoi of prevention, which originated in the important goal of educating the public in the early twentieth century and circulated in different forms later in the century as new information about the causes of different types of cancer led to an emphasis on behaviors that could safeguard against its development. Although all of the cancer topoi discussed previously have some positive features, the medical benefits of cancer prevention are perhaps most evident. Yet, as is the case of the war and positivity topoi, the prevention topos is also permeated with eugenic strains of thought. Certainly arguments for prevention alert people to specific behaviors that significantly increase the risk of cancer, as well as potentially bringing to light environmental issues that need to be addressed on a broader societal level. At the same time, arguments suggesting that cancer can be controlled through appropriate attention to behavior and environment can hold problematic repercussions, as they frequently emphasize control measures that may or may not be successful and are not equally available to everyone. The emphasis on prevention also supports a cultural mandate to assure us that troubling phenomena can be controlled through determined action, usefully drawing our attention away from the intolerable unpredictability of cancer and its capacity to strike people whose illness cannot be accounted for through even the most thorough scrutiny of their lifestyle. Prevention topoi therefore serve as another example of how lines of argument about cancer hold some benefit while tending to reinforce the cultural emphasis on autonomy that assigns responsibility to individuals charged with upholding the standards of normalcy expected by an anxious public. This pattern invokes again the eugenic vision of a world in which particular forms of intelligence, behaviors, and dispositions must be cultivated to ensure the strength of society through ensuring the survival of those members of the population who possess the right qualities.

PURSUING PREVENTION

The history of cancer is defined by a dynamic relationship between the search for effective treatment methods and the effort to identify physical and social factors that cause the disease. While the shame surrounding cancer prior to the twentieth century was not clearly defined, the sense that people might be responsible for their condition connected with an interest in what might bring the disease about. James Patterson discusses the emergence of varied late nineteenth-century theories that suggested possible causes of cancer, including heredity, contagion, stress, and "luxurious living."[1] The twentieth-century notion that rising cancer statistics could be attributed to the conditions of modern life led to the concerted exploration of potential measures that might be taken to lower the risk of cancer, such as exercise and diet.[2]

As discussed previously, the twentieth century saw the development of cancer publicity as a mechanism for informing the public about the importance of early detection, an initiative that connected with efforts to identify potential causes of cancer, including the exploration of varied sources of irritation that might lead to malignancy. The precedence for the focus on irritation as a potential cause of cancer had been established as early as 1775, when Dr. Percivall Pott discovered that frequent exposure to soot had caused a high incidence of scrotal cancer among chimney sweeps.[3] Across the decades of the twentieth century, ongoing advances in laboratory research were accompanied by calls for greater attention not only to the internal cellular causes of cancer but also to the social and environmental conditions that might contribute to the development of the disease. The papers of Frederick L. Hoffman, Prudential Insurance Company statistician and chair of the American Society for the Control of Cancer's Statistics Committee, reflect attention early in the twentieth century to environmental factors that might cause cancer. A document from that collection titled "Note on the Smoke Problem of Pittsburg in its Relation to Cancer" traces historical studies, including a 1906 AMA journal article exploring the effects of coal dust on the lymphatic system, to suggest potential relationships between cancer and various sources of industrial fuel. The article concludes that "the best medical opinion of the world now recognizes that smoke is a direct menace to public health, in that it predisposes the lungs to tuberculosis and pneumonia, as well as other acute diseases, by filling the air with carbon particles which lodge in the lungs, and by causing housekeepers to keep windows and doors closed to keep out the drifting soot."[4] Although acknowledging that there seems to be decisive evidence that smoke is a health hazard, and at the very least interferes with "buoyancy of spirits," the writer argues that there is much that is not yet known about the specific risks associated with environmental causes: "All of these observations confirm the view that there is a distinct relation between the smoke evil and the public health; how far this relation affects the mortality from cancer cannot at the present time be established."[5] Hoffman's statistical review also pointed to the "apparent menace of cancer in the pitch and tar industries," a particular concern in England.[6]

Early efforts to acquire empirical data that indicated causes of cancer were extended in the ensuing decades as researchers expanded their previous focus on internal causes, including genetics, to consider interactions between individuals and the external world. The 1940s saw both an increase in public discourse concerning cancer treatment and considerable speculation about the causes of cancer and strategies for cancer prevention. During the early 1940s, Memorial Hospital announced the distribution of twenty-five thousand copies of "Cancer and Your Home," a pamphlet focused on prevention and early discovery.[7] Nutrition also came under scrutiny during this period. A *New York Herald Tribune* article (ca. 1940) titled "Science: Diet to Prevent Cancer Sought: Doctors Study Added Clew to Chemical Cure: Experiments with Animal Believed Indicating Key, Big-Scale Test Planned" announced the "search for dietary essentials which would enable the body to perform a simple chemical operation altering the substances that cause cancer and destroying their cancer-producing power."[8] While the article is somewhat vague in its depiction of the causes that might be discovered, author John J. O'Neill is nevertheless optimistic about the outcome: "A dozen or more discoveries, no one of them complete in itself and all of them in the field of biological chemistry, have contributed their share to the seemingly well founded hope that this scourge of all living things eventually may be brought under control."[9]

The energetic pursuit of likely causes of cancer is evident in many examples of cancer rhetoric in the early 1940s. A *New York Herald Tribune* article circa 1941 describes efforts to control cancer through stimulating the immune system; a 1941 *Ladies Home Journal* article identifies sun bathing as a skin cancer risk, while a *Modern Science* article the same year warns of the link between cancer and a vitamin A shortage.[10] In contrast, a 1942 article in the Chicago edition of *Hospital Top Buy* suggests that vitamin B may increase the likelihood of cancer.[11] A number of other 1942 articles explore hormonal and dietary links to cancer; although the 1942 *Niagara Falls Gazette* article announcing a higher incidence of stomach cancer in people from Japan describes this discovery simply as "a phenomenon not entirely understood," this study ultimately resulted in a theory that linked stomach cancer to the heavy consumption of smoked fish in the Japanese diet.[12] A 1948 press release quotes Dr. William E. Smith of the Sloan-Kettering Institute and the chair of a newly formed Cancer Prevention Committee as stating that "the constant, heavy pollution of the city's air with soot is an example of a preventable hazard."[13]

By the 1950s researchers had identified a wide range of carcinogens, "including cigarettes, air pollution, asbestos, X-rays, food additives, aniline dyes, and sunlight," a development that led Congress to establish several safety measures aimed at controlling such risks.[14] In addition, various studies conducted by the Sloan Kettering Institute in the late 1950s focused greater attention on internal mechanisms, such as the body's production of steroids, natural defenses, and the synthesis and use of nucleic acids.[15] Ongoing research into cancer's development during this period also generated increasingly sophisticated methods for determining the intricate networks of phenomena that collectively contributed to cancer's development. An October 21, 1959, press release summarizing a speech by Dr. Peyton Rous at a two-day symposium marking the seventy-fifth anniversary of Memorial Center, titled *Toward the Conquest of Cancer*, states that "knowledge of the steps by which cancer develops may be of greater importance than finding out why it develops."[16] At the same symposium, Dr. Robert E. Eckardt, director of the medical research division of the Esso Research and Engineering Company, called for "a 'quantitative approach' to the problem of what causes cancer," emphasizing the need for "the keenest type of impartial judgment" to accompany a careful review of evidence about food safety; Eckardt insists that both carcinogens and those co-carcinogens that accelerate cancer's development should be considered, as slow progress in attending to this area must not "supplant control of exposure to possible cancer-causing agents."[17] The institute's decision to devote more attention to prevention was reinforced in a 1960 announcement by John R. Heller, president of Memorial Sloan-Kettering Cancer Center, and Dr. Frank L. Horsfall Jr., president and director of the Sloan-Kettering Institute for Cancer Research. As described in the press release, Horsfall states that although the center's major objective since it was established in 1945 was treatment and control of cancer, it had recently "accepted as a further important responsibility an additional large program of research, the primary objectives of which are to determine the causes of cancer. Because of the probability that external or environmental factors may contribute to the effects of internal or biological factors which can lead to the development of cancers, both types of potentially related factors are to be investigated as thoroughly as is feasible."[18] Heller notes the importance of acknowledging that varied environmental changes in industrial society might be seen as factors in cancer's development but adds that "only a few external factors are by themselves likely to be direct causative factors."[19]

By the following year, Horsfall was able to announce the discovery that cancer, "no matter what the inducing agent, is ultimately the result of a change in the chromosomal nucleic acid (DNA) of the affected cells," an insight that provided the basis for an "orderly" examination of the complex relationship between external factors and internal responses that ultimately lead to the development of cancer.[20] This insight led to further attention to how the body's internal composition accounts for its response to the external world. A February 15, 1961, press release announced a film series on genetics developed by the Sloan-Kettering Institute's Donald S. Walker Laboratory, while an April 14, 1962, press release announced a study exploring the relationship between aging, decreased immune responses, and the occurrence of cancer.[21] In February 1964, Dr. Leo Wade, vice president for administration of the Sloan-Kettering Institute, delivered an address to the American Academy of Occupational Medicine, titled "Occupation and Cancer." The address attended to the long history of links between cancer and particular types of work, which underscored the relationship between cancer and the environment, an insight that set the stage for arguments promoting action to protect workers from undue exposure to hazardous conditions. Wade asserted that "protective clothing, personal hygiene, nutrition, industrial measures should be exploited to the utmost. The urgency of the problems demands such action." At the same time, Wade warned "against contribution to a solitary environmental factor the ultimate causation of cancer," adding that it is important to study "fundamental processes of the cellular level" in order to understand fully the causes of cancer.[22] The focus on prevention that emerged in the late 1950s and 1960s clearly opened the path to a number of important insights about the complexity of how cancer comes into being.

Much of the public attention to the subject of cancer prevention during the mid-twentieth century focused on smoking. Emerging arguments on this topic underscore persistent tensions between the eugenic goals of moving civilization forward through thriving industries and the need to protect civilization from the negative consequences of unregulated support for corporate interests. Although tobacco was viewed with suspicion as early as the late nineteenth century, the suggested link between tobacco and cancer was controversial in large measure because tobacco was such a profitable industry.[23] For this reason, the relationship between cancer and cigarette smoking was hotly debated during the early decades of the twentieth century. While some researchers in the 1930s were convinced of the link, others disputed this opinion, a view that was of course strongly supported by the tobacco industry.[24] Although the prevalence of smoking in the 1940s was accompanied by a steady rise in lung cancer, it took another decade and a number of definitive research studies to convince most people that the two were in fact connected.[25] Even then, many physicians, scientists, and health policy makers were reluctant to make definite claims about the link. It was only in 1964 that the surgeon general issued a report that clearly articulated the proven connection between smoking and cancer, which set the stage for the Federal Trade Commission's subsequent action to regulate tobacco advertisement.[26]

Developments in cancer prevention are too vast and complex to be thoroughly covered in a single chapter, and it is not within the scope of this book to provide a complete history of specific debates about cancer prevention. Arguments that shaped the evolving public understanding of the link between lung cancer and smoking, alongside concerted efforts of the tobacco industry to challenge that connection, featuring the testimony of cancer researchers employed to support their cause, could constitute a book project in its own right. The purpose of this chapter is not to provide a detailed overview of the history of cancer prevention but to outline a substantial shift in cancer rhetoric that took place as the focus of cancer publicity gradually shifted from early detection to aggressive treatment to prevention, a shift that exacerbated the previous emphasis on the need to take charge of the problem—and the potential to assert control through knowledge.

The heightened interest in prevention that had begun to take root midcentury began a cycle of research that generated suggested preventative measures, with particular attention to the conditions created by industrial production.[27]

This period therefore saw a transition from cancer rhetoric that had been highly focused on individual action to lines of argument that attended to political, economic, and social factors that contributed to cancer's dominant place in modern society. And once again, cancer topoi for prevention acquired greater urgency as the need to assert the value of modern progress functioned in an uneasy tension with evidence that the scientific, military, and industrial advances that made that progress possible might be responsible for increasing the risk of cancer.

This tension led to a doubling down on confident rhetorics of progress, since the alternative of questioning the benefits of modern life would go against firmly inscribed twentieth-century American values. Cancer rhetorics of this period acknowledged that modern advances might have added to the risk factors associated with cancer but at the same time firmly upheld modern advances in science and technology as the path to discovering solutions, including measures that those with adequate knowledge could deploy to discover definitive causes that could lead to the prevention of cancer entirely. A 1971 report on the National Cancer Act makes the bold claim that "we know that cancer is preventable," and that recognition fueled a search for precisely how prevention could be ensured.[28] A 1978 press release announcing a $4 million grant from the Sherman Fairchild Foundation to Memorial Sloan-Kettering outlines a plan to direct significant effort "to study the role of diet and nutrition in immunity and the development of disease."[29] In approximately the same year, Memorial Sloan-Kettering announced the publication of a two-part study titled "The Workplace as a Cause of Cancer," in which Drs. David Schottenfeld and Joanna Hass discovered "some 40 chemicals and physical agents found in the workplace, including wood dust, iron oxides, nickel and lead" as likely causes of cancer.[30] During the 1980s the attention to environmental factors was supplemented by growing interest in nutrition; Olson attributes the National Cancer Institute (NCI)'s awareness of the relationship between cancer and nutrition to Guy Newell, whose attention to this subject led the NCI to acknowledge in the late 1980s that nutrition was "a key element in cancer prevention."[31] The interest in potential causes also led to research that illuminated specific environmental factors that caused particular types of cancer, such as the connection between ultraviolet light and skin cancer.[32] Olson documents the introduction during the 1980s of prevention as "a subdiscipline of oncology" at MD Anderson, a development that came about largely through the influence of Charles A. LeMaistre.[33] Developments focused on the relationship between cancer and chemicals, diet, and stress led to the widespread view that the conditions of modern civilization were largely to blame for what appeared to be cancer's increasing presence during this period, but this recognition was accompanied by a push for behavior modification as a central goal in helping people lower the risk of cancer.[34] Thus, the American emphasis on individualism was deployed to foreground the goal of educating people to pursue measures that could control their circumstances, rather than centering on public health as embedded in larger systemic issues. As S. Lochlann Jain notes, "the focus on awareness and screening does not bring us any closer to understanding the ways that key aspects of the economy involve both causing and treating cancer."[35] The topos of prevention included some arguments focused on a more socially oriented solution to the problem of cancer, but longstanding assumptions about cancer and personal health also continued to be evident. Thus, the threats caused by civilization are offset by a eugenic emphasis on cultivating the characteristics available to "civilized" individuals—intelligent, forward-thinking, and proactive—that will position them to devise strategies for countering the negative features associated with society's progress.

PREVENTION AND "THE CANCER ESTABLISHMENT"

Although research in cancer treatment certainly continued, cancer prevention assumed a more significant role in public discourse about cancer across the latter decades of the century. Of course, attention to cancer prevention holds obvious public health benefits. The surgeon general's warning about the hazards of cigarette smoking, accompanied by warning labels on cigarette packaging and the reduction of tobacco advertising, led to widespread public awareness of the link between smoking and lung cancer, as well as heart disease and emphysema. Other studies focused on potential environmental causes pertaining to cancer also led to concrete measures beneficial to public health, an important step that supplemented the ongoing effort to devise more effective treatments for cancer once it had developed.

The interest in prevention also generated a sense of empowerment and critical awareness about the role individuals could play in protecting public health. This perceived benefit was particularly evident as the work of cancer activists initiated what proved to be a controversial effort to push the central focus of public discourse toward preventive measures that included attention to social systems and away from the established emphasis on early detection and treatment focused on individuals. Much of this controversy was defined by a division between cancer advocates dedicated to pursuing environmental changes that they perceived as certain to contribute to cancer prevention and researchers who were for various reasons not always supportive of those efforts. As previously discussed, it was not the case that cancer researchers were uninterested in cancer prevention; in fact, attention to treatment in major cancer centers was consistently linked with research into potential causes of cancer, and the ASCC articulated both prevention and early detection as key elements of its mission from the time of its founding.

However, cancer researchers did not always demonstrate the strong belief in the efficacy of specific prevention initiatives that advocates hoped for, a gulf that widened as frustration over the ravages of cancer treatment grew and the evidence of environmental factors at times seemed to outpace research that could support an aggressive response to those concerns. One reason for this attitude in the early years of cancer research was the widespread opinion of medical researchers that the questions surrounding prevention were extremely complex and difficult to determine with any certainty. A 1942 article in the *Birmingham Post* quoted Memorial Hospital director Cornelius P. Rhoads as advancing the view that a cancer cure might be achieved before the discovery of its cause, which reflected the assumption that efforts to pinpoint causes were constantly shifting and shaped by a multitude of contingencies.[36]

The awareness of the challenges surrounding research into cancer prevention led many scientists to be understandably wary of the zeal to make certain claims about the environmental causes of cancer. Tension between reputable cancer researchers and upstarts promising certain knowledge about cancer was certainly nothing new. In a 1915 letter to Curtis E. Lakeman, Frederick L. Hoffman writes, "You have probably seen the cancer article in the New York Sun, main section, Sunday, November 14th, regarding another cancer cure. It seems to me that at the next meeting of the Committee it might be well to adopt a circular letter to the editorial staff of the principal daily newspapers protesting against the elaborate and conspicuous publication of alleged cancer cures to the great detriment to the cause of cancer control and the serious injury to the public at large."[37] Uninformed opinions about causes of cancer were at least as prolific as suggested cures. As a statistician, Hoffman was alert to differences between evidence and conjecture. A letter to Lakeman dated January 26, 1915, disputes the claim to a parallel statistical increase in cancer and appendicitis, insisting that there is in fact no statistical relationship between the two.[38]

As discussed in chapter 1, the increase in cancer publicity over the course of the century held hazards as well as benefits. The goal of informing the public and encouraging action in support of the early detection and prevention of cancer often included emotional appeals that departed from what cancer researchers considered to be a factual representation of the evidence at hand. Frank Horsfall's 1960 letter to John Heller protesting the "Cancer Virus Script" that NBC shared with Memorial Sloan-Kettering, referenced in chapter 1, focused on the program's failure to be strictly accurate in its discussion of the potential causes of leukemia: "The implied suggestion that leukemia is infectious and contagious is both regrettable and hazardous. Much of what is said is obviously bald speculation without basis in fact but the impact on the public will have the effect of making them think that knowledge is far ahead of its present state."[39] It is unsurprising that media devoted to providing the public with information, particularly in an area where certainty was desperately longed for, would at times find it difficult to manage the complexity of cancer research and the slow pace at which news was available.

Just as the widespread concern about cancer and the impatience to find alternative treatments contributed to interest in the promise that psychology could promote healing through supporting a positive mental state, so the focus on prevention generated a robust public discussion that supplemented and at times directly challenged mainstream cancer research. Richard G. Berger, a research chemist and early proponent of prevention, launched a rhetorical campaign in the late 1930s in support of aggressive measures to control industrial activity that he considered to be responsible for increasing cancer rates. Berger's dedication to his cause included the establishment of an organization, Cancer Prevention, Inc., which had the stated purpose of publicizing possible causes of cancer and advocating for prevention efforts. A 1950 article in *Nature's Path* titled "Prevent Cancer!" outlines the basic premises of Berger's argument, which was persistently advanced through numerous handbills distributed to the public free of charge, as well as via magazine articles and letters to the editor. Early in the article, Berger succinctly states his claim: "I have maintained, consistently, that cancer can be prevented at insignificant cost, as a long-range proposition, by reduction of our carcinogenic (cancer-causing) contacts." Berger charges that soot, which "is in the smoky air we breathe and on much of the food we eat," holds particular dangers to public health: "*Because of its high cancer-causing tar content, this soot is probably the leading cause of cancer today*" (emphasis in the original). But Berger's attention does not rest solely with soot; he also makes note of the four hundred cancer-causing chemicals referenced but not fully discussed in the Connecticut Cancer Society's "1950 Report of Progress" and launches extensive criticism of the lack of attention to other cancer risks, including tobacco smoking, arsenic from insecticide sprays, x-ray exposure, and the coal tar spread on roads.[40]

Berger's arguments for cancer prevention adopted a combative tone consonant with later public prevention arguments. Berger repeatedly charges those who should be at the forefront in protecting public health with failure to do their duty. In his view, the fact "that cancer will kill horribly and unnecessarily at least 20 million Americans now alive" is the result of inaction on the part of the cancer industry, which in his view is too heavily embroiled in corporate interests to maintain an appropriate focus on human life: "The arch crime against modern civilization is the fact that *the public is not being informed by our scientists, cancer societies, memorial funds, or life insurance companies about dangerous cancer-causing irritants abundant in our daily living*" (emphasis original). He pulls no punches in attributing the blame for this failure on individual and corporate greed: "There's big money for some in this gruesome debacle because hundreds of surgeons and radiologists specializing in cancer have gross incomes from fifty to several hundred thousand dollars per year. At the same time I know of no one striving for cancer prevention who derives any income therefrom." Philanthropic cancer agencies are also subject to Berger's critical scrutiny: "The cancer societies and memorial funds which collect millions of dollars from the public every year DON'T tell you about the following abundant dangerous carcinogens. (Such publicity interferes with some businesses)."[41] This provocative claim is restated in various venues; Berger's late 1940s pamphlet "Arrest Cancer, (Why Not?) It's Wanted for Murder!" argues that "anti-cancer organizations appeal for donations, while refraining from publicizing the deadly cancer-causing irritants in daily civilized living," a strategy that "is expedient in the solicitation of contributions, because no one (especially no sponsors or advertisers) can be offended." Berger goes on to suggest that cancer organizations are therefore complicit in the prevalence of cancer in modern life: "The immense sums of money collected are invariably used to augment the same type of organizations and procedures which have failed to halt the inexorable increase of cancer in the past."[42] A February 1951 *Nature's Path* column explicitly charges the American Cancer Society with failure to be aggressive in publicizing the dangers of tobacco smoking, urging the group to shift its focus from detection to prevention.[43]

Although Berger operated on the fringes of public debate over the course of several decades, his suggestion that cancer researchers and advocacy groups were part of the problem was sufficiently controversial to cause a measure of discomfort. A brief 1950 *California Farmer* column describing Berger's work predicts the "uproar the acceptance of this theory could produce," as "the doctors who spend much of their time testing and endorsing cigarettes, if we are to believe the radio, might have to give up smoking." The column goes on to say, "You can readily see what an irritant Berger is to a lot of commercial companies who handle various suspect products."[44] Copies of a number of Berger's columns and handbills can be found in Mary Lasker's papers, which suggests that the ACS leaders took note of his claims, and in 1954 the organization was compelled to write a memo in response to the widespread circulation of materials from Cancer Prevention, Inc. to various cancer organizations, including branches of the ACS. The memo notes that Berger's organization has been "largely a one-man operation, and its activities have been confined to disseminating Mr. Berger's theories, rather than to conducting research as the name would indicate." While acknowledging that Berger has some credibility as an MIT chemistry graduate and praising his "honesty and integrity," the memo goes on to state, "His 'research' activities have been in the nature of a hobby. He is said to be a sincere, well-meaning but overly-enthusiastic individual who pursues his strong convictions concerning the causes and prevention of cancer in an unscientific manner."[45] In spite of the ACS's apparent appreciation for Berger's sincerity, the use of sneer quotes around the word research, coupled with the dismissal of the "unscientific manner" with which he conducts his work, clearly conveyed the organization's frustration with Berger's attacks, reinforcing the *California Farmer*'s suggestion that "Mr. Berger is likely to produce many stomach ulcers."[46]

Whatever the limitations of Berger's "one-man operation" may have been, he was not inaccurate in suggesting that even well-meaning institutions have complicated motives and loyalties, as well as a vexed relationship with standards of American social improvement that have historically been tied to profit. The basic outlines of this argument proved to be increasingly significant in the latter decades of the century. The links between cancer research and the military industrial complex, as described in chapter 2, contributed to growing suspicion from various sides concerning the complicity of "the cancer establishment" in overlooking environmental causes. In addition to a legacy tarnished by his connection to eugenics, ACS director Clarence Cook Little was repeatedly attacked during this period for his reluctance to accept evidence pertaining to the link between smoking and lung cancer, an attitude that critics attributed to close ties to the tobacco industry, including service on the Board of the Tobacco Industry Research Committee. Such suspicions continued to escalate in subsequent decades, as journalists and activist groups such as the Breast Cancer Prevention Collaborative Research Group also pointed to conflicts of interest that prevented cancer researchers from being as aggressive as they should be in investigating other links between cancer and industry. Olson summarizes the political climate during this period: "Cancer politics had come full circle. In the 1950s and 1960s right-wing critics of American medicine, such as the John Birch Society, had accused physicians and hospitals of concealing potential cancer cures in order to jack up fees. A cure for cancer would put the cancer establishment out of business. Now, in the 1980s and 1990s, left-wing ideologues disparaged cancer practitioners for exactly the same reason, accusing them of ignoring cancer prevention in order to line their pockets."[47]

One influential voice in efforts to advance cancer prevention as a political cause in the latter decades of the century was that of Samuel S. Epstein, cancer researcher, public health faculty member, and president of the Rachel Carson Trust. Epstein's 1979 book *The Politics of Cancer* provided an overview of current research pointing to environmental causes of cancer, as well as offering a critical perspective on the reasons the links between cancer and the environment had not been consistently investigated by the cancer establishment. Epstein maintains that "an informed consensus has gradually developed that most cancer is environmental in origin and is therefore preventable" but argues that various factors have interfered with the persistent investigation of causes that might be addressed.[48] Some of these factors can be categorized as negligence; Epstein notes that Congress, various federal agencies, and the NCI were for many decades so thoroughly focused on the promise of a cancer cure that they had little time to spare for the subject of prevention.[49] But Epstein also argues that external issues interfered with attention to prevention. He acknowledges that causes of cancer are often difficult to determine scientifically and notes that further complications arise when science is connected with economic interests. He goes on to argue that the costs of addressing environmental hazards are high, and cancer researchers and agencies have often been supported by industries whose interests do not align with the significant financial investment needed to change the status quo. Epstein provides a thorough critique of the conflicts of interest that prevented cancer agencies such as the NCI and advocacy groups such as the ACS from attending to what he considered to be the evident links between cancer and substances such as industrial chemicals. Epstein charges that "the low priority which the NCI has accorded to research on environmental carcinogenesis in the past has been an important factor in limiting possible regulatory initiatives for cancer prevention and control" and calls for a political approach that goes beyond "scientific effort or individual action."[50]

Feminist voices played a particularly significant role in taking up Epstein's call as the century moved forward. While much of Rose Kushner's breast cancer memoir focuses on how her personal experience can help women make informed decisions about their treatment options, she establishes a substantial foundation for breast cancer activism in a chapter devoted to the "why" of breast cancer. This topic leads her to discuss what she considers to be the unacknowledged dangers of oral contraceptives, which in her view should be more thoroughly investigated and documented for the dangers they present to women's health. Kushner indirectly responds to her own question, "Who can understand the FDA?" with a brief discussion of the personal and political ties between Warner-Lambert founder Elmer H. Bobst and Richard Nixon as well as a reference to FDA leaders, who are for the most part medical professionals and scientists who nevertheless have a "business outlook."[51] Audre Lorde is even more pointed in connecting her breast cancer diagnosis to environmental causes that she and others must combat: "For me, my scars are an honorable reminder that I may be a casualty in the cosmic war against radiation, animal fat, air pollution, McDonald's hamburgers, and Red Dye No. 2, but the fight is still going on, and I am still a part of it."[52] Kushner, Lorde, and Epstein set the stage for later arguments that advances in cancer research are constrained by business interests in varied and problematic ways, and they also provided models for rhetorics of cancer activism launched by people with cancer.

These seminal arguments were followed by an increasingly powerful wave of cancer activism in the 1980s and 1990s. Lisa Diedrich writes, "I take 1980 to mark the emergence of a new figure—the political patient—and a new genre—the patient's counternarrative to medical discourse as exemplified by doctors' charts and case histories."[53] Although cancer patients had begun speaking and writing about their experiences decades earlier, the era of the politicized patient, empowered to speak about their experiences and to play an active role in seeking answers about cancer's causes and treatments, sets the stage for the emergence of breast cancer activism as a movement in the 1990s, a movement anticipated in the 1985 establishment of Breast Cancer Awareness Month and marked by the 1991 establishment of the National Breast Cancer Coalition.[54] This environment of activism is captured in a 1993 special issue of *Ms.* magazine titled "The Politics of Breast Cancer." The lead article in the magazine, Susan Rennie's "Breast Cancer Prevention: Diet vs. Drugs," celebrates the fact that "women, taking their cue from AIDS activists, have also begun to 'act up,' by organizing, demonstrating, agitating, and lobbying" to pursue more effective approaches to breast cancer prevention and treatment.[55] Rennie maintains that the link between diet and breast cancer needs to be more thoroughly considered, as do environmental and hormonal factors, but charges that "the National Cancer Institute (NCI), backed up by its powerful nongovernmental ally, the American Cancer Society, has relegated breast cancer prevention to funding scraps left over from the therapy research feeding trough."[56] She insists that women should "not tolerate any subversion of the only ongoing investigation into the role of dietary fat because policymakers like NCAB [National Cancer Advisory Board] chair David Korn have decided that we might not be able to do what is good for us."[57]

The same issue features an article by Liane Clorfene-Casten that extensively discusses environmental connections to breast cancer. Clorfene-Casten argues for the need "to refocus the dialogue and the agenda" away from previous warnings about "hereditary, biological, and behavioral factors that increase our risk of developing breast cancer."[58] After raising the question "What would happen to both mortality and incidence rates if all known carcinogenic organochlorines were totally banned from the environment?" Clorfene-Casten goes on to cite Epstein in asking why the ACS and "the rest of the cancer establishment" have participated in "blame-the-victim theories" rather than pursuing answers concerning environmental causes of cancer and pressing for the elimination of those features of modern life.[59] Clorfene-Casten's article is followed by a brief addendum that describes ways in which the "mostly male establishment" (comprising the NCI, ACS, and Memorial Sloan Kettering Cancer Center) that sets priorities for cancer research has created "a golden circle of power and money, where many of the key players are connected."[60] In her view, this "golden circle" accounts for the overwhelming emphasis on business interests that benefit from the promulgation of expensive cancer treatments and would suffer from the elimination of environmental carcinogenics that serve the needs of industry. The *Ms.* special issue reflects the central role of feminists in the progression of cancer activism, signaling a growing interest in grass-roots efforts to heighten awareness of breast cancer and offer women alternatives to the course of treatment offered by the "mostly male establishment." Four years later, a *Ms.* issue featured an article on the World Conference on Breast Cancer, an event that brought together 650 delegates around the world to create a network of feminist activism focused on breast cancer awareness. Michele Landsberg's account emphasizes the ways in which the conference broke the "corporate, media, and government silence" that had prohibited knowledge about the environmental causes of breast cancer. Landsberg challenges mainstream media accounts that depicted the conference as "simplistic or confrontational," adding that "to be able to sneer at feminists and ridicule their concerns is an effective diversionary tactic to protect transnational corporations from their most dangerous enemy: a public roused to anger over environmental degradation."[61] By the late 1990s, the angry public, led by people with cancer, had assumed a new role in the promulgation of cancer rhetorics that challenged previous patterns of situating the problem firmly within the bodies, minds, and emotions of individuals with cancer.

There is certainly value in public arguments pressing the medical community to be more aggressive in acknowledging the significant relationship between cancer and the environment. At the same time, historical records document the struggles early cancer researchers interested in exploring environmental factors in cancer's development faced as they sought to determine the precise role of the environment alongside other risk factors that might affect the health of individuals. Meanwhile, the rapid proliferation of public arguments concerning possible environmental factors at times prompted highly speculative conclusions, an issue that led to the 1979 publication of an NCI pamphlet titled "Everything Doesn't Cause Cancer."[62] Cancer researchers also faced the challenge of determining the exact point at which evidence pertaining to environmental factors justifies policy decisions. The October 19, 1959, press release describing an address at the "Toward the Conquest of Cancer" symposium delivered by Dr. Paul Steiner, a researcher at the Philadelphia Institute for Cancer Research and University of Pennsylvania School of Medicine, begins with the question, "How can knowledge on cancer prevention most effectively be applied under a democratic system?" While Steiner's address demonstrates keen interest in cancer prevention, he also raises important questions about the role of education and legislation in determining steps that should be taken to protect public health. Steiner predicts that "the prevention of cancer, now practiced on a small scale, will become possible in the major types if cancer-causing agents become recognized and abolished," but he also raises questions pertaining to the amount of evidence needed "to embark upon large scale preventive programs."[63] While Berger and the cancer activists who followed him were certainly accurate in making note of the difficulty of separating the funding needs of medical research from corporate interests, arguments put forward by cancer researchers point to the challenges of finding an appropriate balance among the complexities of scientific inquiry and standards of evidence, the values of democracy and free enterprise, and urgent public health priorities.

At the same time, these issues reflect an ongoing tension that is at work in the circulation of all public cancer rhetoric, which comes from the need to create appeals for education and research support that will resonate with audiences who are influenced by long-standing constraints that include the importance of medical research, appreciation for scientific advances, and a genuine concern for public health, but also engage with commitments to capitalism and profit, eugenic ideologies, social assumptions embedded in economic privilege and ableism, and faith in progress at all costs. The people created by cancer topoi are therefore a complicated blend of hopes and fears, a dynamic reflected in lines of argument that emphasize the worthy aims of prevention, the fears of going too far in undermining industry, and the assurance that social improvement is possible and should be pursued no matter what the cost.

PREVENTION, EUGENICS, AND THE IDEAL CANCER PATIENT

Although cancer prevention topoi at times provide helpful avenues for personal agency in matters pertaining to public health, the emphasis on behavior as a feature of prevention reinforces public assumptions that the dangers of cancer can be diminished by the idealized image of an individual capable of taking charge of the public health menace. The irony underlying this ideal is that it projects a person whose path to good health depends upon constant attention to the likelihood of illness. While acknowledging that uses of medical technologies have saved lives, Maren Klawiter notes the complications that arise from measures that turn "asymptomatic women into risky subjects."[64] The benefits available through aggressive diagnostic measures such as mammography and the PSA have been debated, as have the appropriate target populations for these tests.[65] Although some of the evidence concerning environmental impacts on cancer has been compelling, other speculations about the links between cancer and specific environmental factors and behaviors have been less definitive, while drastic measures to preempt the potential development of cancer through surgical procedures have been fraught with controversy.

As has been shown in previous chapters, efforts to assert control over cancer place the people called into being by cancer rhetoric in a challenging position. The call to mount a courageous battle against cancer, to demonstrate cheerfulness in the face of adversity, and to seize control of one's health all have some merit, but they also impose pressure on those whose circumstances make it difficult if not impossible to participate in "the realm of the normal" that these lines of argument often seek to uphold.[66] The assumption that the control of cancer is within the individual's grasp also might suggest that those who are not capable of preventive measures are somehow deficient. The conclusion of Clarence Little's "Cancer Can Be Cured," a circa 1940 article pertaining to the importance of cancer awareness, includes the statement, "Individual intelligence, courage, and promptness mean the control of cancer."[67] While these words might be interpreted as inspiring, they also imply that when cancer is not controlled, it is due to the absence of these meritorious qualities in the individual.

Moreover, the promise of acquiring control over cancer is certainly more within the grasp of some people than others, and the social and economic privilege attached to much twentieth-century cancer advocacy cannot go unnoticed. Walter Ross's history of the ACS includes the recognition that the founders of the ASCC were white men and that the organization remained "a kind of Caucasian club" for several decades.[68] Change came to the organization through attention to community outreach during the 1960s, led in Washington, DC, by a young African American oncologist named Lasalle D. Leffall Jr., whose election as president of the DC division coincided with important findings concerning cancer mortality rates in the African American community. Dr. Leffall's prominent role in the organization coincided with the appointment of the ACS's first African American executive staff member, News Editor John Henry Jones.[69]

While the increasing inclusion of members of underrepresented groups in leadership positions within the ACS over the latter portion of the twentieth century is noteworthy, it is nevertheless difficult to avoid the rhetorical strains that in effect constitute a people who are participants in "a kind of Caucasian club." In part, this can be explained by the fact that cancer advocacy organizations such as the ASCC began during a period when the ability to engage public attention was tied to the influence and wealth that rested almost entirely in white society. In his 1913 address delivered before the National Conference of Charities and Correction, Curtis E. Lakeman explains that the formation of the ASCC began with medical professionals who soon reached the conclusion that a movement intended largely for the instruction and benefit of the laity should be organized and directed to a considerable extent by men and women outside the medical profession, although in the closest cooperation with the best available medical experts. Accordingly, the committee invited to its preliminary meetings a number of experienced and influential men and women who were especially interested in the cancer problem. Five of these public-spirited citizens guaranteed the first year's expenses of the proposed organization to the amount of $5000, on the condition that its plan and purpose should meet with the approval of the medical profession as a whole.[70]

Accompanying the knowledge that wealthy white people would be most likely to have access to the capital and influence that would provide access to medical professionals and leverage public attention was the understanding that arguments appealing to economic concerns conceived as relevant to a prosperous white community would garner further support. Lakeman's description of strategies employed to spark interest in the social problem of cancer includes an emphasis on statistical information and an appeal to the presidents of insurance companies, who were bound to have particular interest in "a movement which, in course of time, would certainly prove of advantage to their policyholders."[71] Thus the use of statistics to establish authority, discussed in chapter 1, also constituted an audience interested in the type of demographic information these statistics provided.

As discussed previously, the ASCC's focus on gathering information that would educate the public yielded a strong emphasis on logical arguments filled with statistical information. Frederick Hoffman's strategic use of statistics not only ensured that the organization was well positioned to gather data pertinent to acquiring a more thorough understanding of cancer but also persistently tied the search to understand and prevent cancer to the concerns of insurance companies. Hoffman's article titled "The Statistical Evidence of the Increase in Cancer" does explicitly attend to the issue of race in relation to cancer, with particular attention to the change in cancer rates among Black people after slavery: "The importance of the race factor is illustrated by a study of the records of thirty southern cities where the cancer death rate among Whites was 80.3 per 100,000 of population and 55.2 for the colored. There has been a considerable increase in the negro cancer death rate since the Civil War, especially marked in the case of cancer of the uterus. As far as the data can be relied upon cancer is extremely rare among native American races, such as the North American Indian, the Esquimo and the Negroes of the West Indies. There would indeed seem to be a very close relation between cancer frequency and the degree of material civilization."[72]

The link between cancer and civilization undermined eugenic optimism concerning the certain progress available through modern society's production and economic advancement. Although they did not directly acknowledge this conflict, Hoffman and others rhetorically framed the statistical link between cancer and civilization as an economic danger that would enlist the interest of insurance companies and business leaders. Lakeman's "Cancer as a

Social Problem" address frames the importance of cancer research as based in part on its social and economic impact:

> Only an elementary consideration of the foregoing statistics is required in order to visualize the terrific onslaught of cancer against men and women at the most useful period of life and at the age when the care and guidance of children and the discharge of business responsibilities make the mother and father most valuable to society. Cancer is therefore a deadly force in the destruction of homes. . . . The life insurance companies realize the significance of cancer to utmost. As Mr. Edward A. Woods of Pittsburgh recently pointed out cancer attacks the very class of persons most largely insured. The disease is more prevalent if anything among well to do civilized people living under sanitary conditions. Its onset cannot be foreseen or detected through physique, hereditary or environment as is the case with tuberculosis and other diseases. For these reasons cancer increases the cost of life insurance for which we in America pay nearly a billion dollars annually.[73]

The theme of cancer as a problem worth noting due to its prevalence among those who are contributors to society was further emphasized by Hoffman in a 1914 letter in which he recommended changes to an article Lakeman was writing about cancer. Hoffman's suggested changes included substituting one of Lakeman's drafted paragraphs with one that provided an explicit portrait of the cancer patient as worthy of concern due to being a prominent member of society:

> Cancer being distinctly a disease of adult life, it is also apparently peculiarly an affliction of the prosperous and well-to-do. Life insurance experience has shown that cancer is more common among persons overweight than among those below the normal weight. Cancer is, therefore, of special interest to insurance companies, and more so in view of the fact that latent evidences of the disease are disclosed with difficulty even by the most rigid medical examinations. Cancer is less prevalent among the class of people generally not insured—that is, the very poor, the mentally afflicted, the primitive races, and the people living under unsanitary conditions. The cancer death rate does not appear to be affected by

> improvements in sanitation. In other words, cancer is exceptionally common among the element considered more desirable for Ordinary life insurance purposes.[74]

This assessment does not engage with obvious questions pertaining to other factors that might account for these statistics, including the possibility that those "generally not insured" lack access to the medical care that would lead to a cancer diagnosis, or that "the very poor, the mentally afflicted" might have health conditions that would lead to death from causes other than cancer. The premise that cancer is "distinctly a disease of adult life" also completely ignores the fact that children do get cancer. These omissions suggest a strategic decision to highlight factors that were deemed likely to garner attention and support for the cause: cancer's role in diminishing society's progress and productivity. As discussed previously, the fact that concerns about diverse populations and age groups are not raised, along with the perception that cancer functions as "peculiarly an affliction of the prosperous and well-to-do," engages the interest of the business community with the means to support cancer research through pointing to cancer as a disease that defies prominent eugenic assumptions concerning the relationship among civilization, health, and strength. This anxiety continues to be evident in cancer rhetoric's evolution in the following decades, and the emergence of prevention topoi helps to shape the imagined persona of the prosperous cancer patient, who is paradoxically more vulnerable but also more capable of adopting prevention measures that can control the threat created by that prosperity. This line of argument sustains the pattern that emerges in the war metaphor and topoi emphasizing the value of positivity in reversing the threat of cancer. The promise of control is particularly evident in arguments surrounding prevention, which often rely on the expectation that if people are only educated enough, smart enough, and careful enough, they can escape cancer entirely. As is the case with other cancer topoi, the difficulty with the promise of control begins with the fact that absolute control of cancer is never possible, no matter how much courage, hopefulness, or intelligence someone possesses. Arguments for prevention involve the further complication of assuming a degree of personal choice that is simply not within the grasp of a large percentage of the population.

One example of the rhetorical construction of an idealized cancer patient shaped by eugenic images appears in a 1944 *Reader's Digest* article (condensed from the health magazine *Hygeia*) titled "An Ounce of Prevention: Today's Cure for Cancer." The snapshot of the visitor to the prevention clinic contains a number of details that reflect eugenic assumptions concerning the qualities that make it possible to overcome the dangers of cancer: "Mrs. W. stepped down happily from the examining table. An attractive woman in her late 30's, this mother of two children looked the picture of health—and she intended to stay that way. Twice a year she went to the cancer prevention clinic for an examination; this was her tenth. Her mother and her mother's mother were struck down by cancer; Mrs. W. need not be."[75] Although the emphasis on Mrs. W.'s attractiveness and the privileges that have given her access to health care are presented alongside the vulnerability that is reflected in her health history, this story underscores the promise of prevention, which in this case converges with early detection. Although Mrs. W.'s family history is bleak, medical progress and Mrs. W.'s diligence have enabled her to escape the fate of her mother and grandmother. Mrs. W.'s attractiveness, marital status, and motherhood, along with the assurance of scientific progress, are subtly woven into the claim that she can achieve control over her unfortunate heredity. The article also summons readers whose ready identification with Mrs. W. will prompt active attention to their health.

A similar rhetorical strategy is used in episode two of *The Endless Frontier*, a 1952 radio series hosted by Raymond Massey. The episode, titled "The Search," features vignettes that depict the positive outcomes experienced by patients who adopt an aggressive approach to health care. The scene featuring "Mrs. Welch" begins with her question: "You . . . you mean I don't have to worry about it anymore, Doctor?," which yields the assurance, "In the majority of cases—no, Mrs. Welch. You see, you caught it in plenty of time."[76]

The representation of attractive women who escape cancer through intelligence and health awareness is also carried forward in a 1965 *American Cancer Society News* article written by Barbara Heimann, Miss American Teen-Ager of 1964, titled "Why I Don't Smoke." Heimann begins the article by noting her discovery that most contestants in the Miss American Teen-Ager competition did not smoke, which also underscores the persistent link between personal appearance, economic privilege, and the ability to resist the dangers of smoking. And, in fact, Heimann highlights the disgusting aesthetic consequences of smoking as much as she does the health risk. Heimann does not demonstrate the health intelligence that Clarence Little promotes,[77] but she does have access to other middle-class orientations that will serve her well in protecting her health. Heimann acknowledges that "exactly how it affects the lungs I cannot say," but she does assert that tobacco "does a lot of harm," presumably knowledge she has absorbed and chosen to act upon. Heimann provides more graphic detail about other negative consequences of smoking in the following paragraph: "Aside from health, smoking means messy ash trays all over the house and in cars, yellow fingers, bad breath, smell of cigarettes on clothing. I don't like these." Although she admits that some of her friends smoke, she makes special note of smoking as a social disadvantage for women: "Contrary to popular belief—and although they don't usually say so—most young men would rather their dates didn't smoke. They still want their girls to act like girls and not puff on tobacco." Thus, the goal of prevention is portrayed not only as a healthy option but also the means for maintaining the norms of middle-class sensibility, including the avoidance of undesirable odors, maintaining white skin untainted by tobacco, and protecting one's desirability as a date. Heimann also adheres to the eugenic "fitter family" mentality, as she acknowledges that her ability to resist the temptation to smoke has at least in part come from the good fortune of her upbringing in a family in which neither her mother nor brothers (one of whom was at West Point and the other at Williams College) smoked. She explains that although her Danish father did smoke, he kept his habit in moderation, with a preference for "pipes and cigars—as most vikings do." In addition to positive family influence, Heimann credits her avoidance of smoking to willpower: "I say that thinking and trying to remember all the bad things connected with smoking could do a lot to help one decide not to smoke. I also suggest that if someone really wants to cut it out, or at least cut down, all she or he has to do is to try to think of one good reason for lighting a cigarette before they do it. Certainly, it could be a better world if we all should try to do the right things and a cleaner and healthier world if everybody stopped smoking."[78]

Heimann's short article highlights the subtle ways in which arguments for prevention are embedded in appeals shaped by eugenic perspectives, as the opportunity to offset the danger of cancer comes from strength of will, intelligence, education, family background, whiteness, citizenship, and a commitment to a version of success focused on adhering to established social and gender roles. This line of reasoning circulates from earlier arguments established in the formation of the ASCC, as illustrated in a speech referenced in chapter 1, "Cancer a Controllable Disease," by Dr. Edward Reynolds, delivered on behalf of the ASCC's Boston Local Committee to the Massachusetts State Federation of Women's Clubs. The basis for Reynolds's argument is that the audience's superior intelligence, gender, and social standing provides them with a unique opportunity for playing a positive role in public health efforts: "You ladies represent an enormous number of women who have been in effect automatically selected from the community as the possessors of intelligence and public spirit. The matter which we wish to bring before you is one which is of interest to both sexes and which must be taken up by both sexes, but it is perhaps of even greater interest to women than to men, and moreover in this, as in so many other movements, the community depends primarily on the keener sympathies of women, on their more active public spirit, and incidentally upon the greater aggregate of time which upon the average they are able and willing to devote to public work, as compared with men."[79] Although Reynolds assures the women that "this mortality is for the most part preventable," he charges them as "picked representatives of an intelligent body" with the task of helping to find appropriate language for "speaking to the less intelligent."[80] Thus, longstanding assumptions concerning race and gender are invoked in imagining an audience of white women who have a particular capacity for sympathy, nurturing and supporting others, and practical intelligence. An additional qualification lies in the fact that the limitations associated with their gender and the privilege available as a result of their race and class have provided them with ample time to engage in volunteer work.

While arguments that encourage early detection and prevention have benefited public health in many ways, the view that prevention can be easily achieved and that education and intelligence equip people to take advantage of this opportunity leads to strains of argument that are more troubling. The increase in publicity about cancer and scientific knowledge also leads to urgent calls for prevention, with the occasional implication that those individuals who are not able to pursue this goal hold some blame for their fate. A 1966 booklet published by the US Department of Health, Education and Welfare describes how educational efforts have substantially improved the prognosis for uterine, breast, and colorectal cancer, but adds, "But learning the facts of cancer is not enough; in order to be saved, people must accept the individual responsibility to act on what they know. Perhaps this can be expressed more clearly in relation to smoking and health. Millions of Americans now know that smoking cigarettes is hazardous, that it causes lung cancer. Smokers know they should quit, but they don't. They do not act on what they know."[81]

While the decision not to smoke could well be classified as an opportunity to exercise individual responsibility, the topos of cancer prevention as an exercise in autonomy becomes a slippery slope, as it contributes to the creation of a people whose outlook on cancer tilts toward particular assumptions about the qualities that allow people to overcome cancer. Although conscientious attention to health is a positive quality, the framing of appeals for prevention, aligned with longstanding eugenic patterns of identifying those flaws responsible for social decline, often shifts into blaming those whose cancer diagnosis might reflect less scrupulous health habits or other undesirable qualities. In their study of how perceptions of the health habits of individuals with cancer shape the emotional responses of observers, Catherine E. Mosher and Sharon Danoff-Burg note that "feelings of pity arise if an observer attributes an illness to uncontrollable factors (e.g., genetics); pity, in turn, increases willingness to help the person. Conversely, if an illness is attributed to controllable factors (e.g., poor health habits), feelings of anger arise that, in turn, evoke neglect of the affected individual."[82] Mosher and Danoff-Burg's study explores the ways in which gender and the perception of controllability influence the responses people have toward those diagnosed with lung cancer; their findings suggest that "cancer-related stigma is a complex phenomenon that may initially be influenced by gender norms and the smoking history of the person with cancer."[83] When the emphasis on individual responsibility is imposed on others, unfortunate consequences arise for those who have been diagnosed with cancer.

Moreover, individual responsibility only goes so far in cancer prevention: many smokers never develop lung disease, and people can develop lung cancer without ever having smoked cigarettes. One interesting consequence of prevention arguments I have noted through the years is the number of people who feel compelled to point out that their loved ones diagnosed with lung cancer never smoked, as though health history and behavior determine one's eligibility for a sympathetic response. Individuals also have limited choice in shaping the environments in which they live and work, which means that arguments for prevention often promise a measure of control that is not as certain as often implied. As discussed previously, Memorial Sloan Kettering's 1948 press release announcing the formation of the Cancer Prevention Committee quotes Dr. William E. Smith of the Sloan-Kettering Institute as identifying soot as "an example of a preventable hazard." Smith also notes that "a great deal of cancer prevention depends not on medical means, but on engineering procedures and public awareness of the need for preventing contact with cancer-producing chemicals."[84] While soot might indeed be preventable, the unanswered question in this and other cases of environmental hazard is, "Preventable by whom?" For most people, the question of precisely how to avoid "cancer-producing chemicals" is a perplexing one. The seemingly straightforward goal of breathing clean air proves to be more elusive than it might appear, particularly for people whose social and economic circumstances limit their options for places to live and work. Certainly advocating for broader environmental reforms is a valuable response, as cancer activists at the end of the century have realized. However, it is important to recognize ways in which varied forms of argument for prevention instead emphasize personal responsibility in managing the hazards that surround us, reflecting a eugenic assumption that inferior biological strains and poor choices account for many of the problems people face.

Despite these evident problems with the promise of prevention arguments, cancer's uncontrollability and defiance of eugenic expectations concerning the strength of the "prosperous and well-to-do" exacerbate the cultural need for assurance that cancer can be tamed; prevention topoi provide a compelling response to this need. The focus on control and personal responsibility often overwhelms the positive value to the public that comes from the identification of risk factors. Susan Yadlon notes that the circulation of breast cancer risk factors in the media typically centers upon diet and reproduction, which "are represented as controllable behaviors: one can alter one's diet and 'plan' childbearing: but there is little one can do about family history, age, or the onset of menses and menopause."[85] Yadlon acknowledges that "the emphasis on individual responsibility and choice" is a common strain in discourse about medicine but argues that both scientific and activist discourses about breast cancer prevention have particular gendered implications, as "breast cancer discourse tacitly (and sometimes not so tacitly) implies that the way to prevent the disease is to follow dominant codes of femininity."[86]

Yet even those who acknowledge that complete control is not possible often imply that knowledge about cancer is in itself a source of power, a statement that has become a staple in recent arguments for genetic testing. Early ideas about the personal and social responsibility required of people with intelligence and education continue to play out in contemporary arguments about diagnostic biotechnologies. In their analysis of the Myriad public marketing campaign for BRACAnalysis, a product that detects genetic mutations associated with reproductive cancers, Zoltan P. Majdik and Carrie Anne Platt note that Myriad's campaign "rhetorically constructs this semblance of autonomous, empowered medical choice by transforming applied genetics' promise of personal empowerment into a personal and familial obligation."[87] The consequence is the creation of "a problematic second persona: a particular (and peculiar) subject position that enables and disables certain ways of acting and making choices, inviting people into a paradoxical position where their medical empowerment becomes predicated on and gives rise to obligations to the self and others."[88] In discussing the ethical complexities surrounding the campaign, Majdik and Platt point out that whether one develops ovarian or breast cancer may or may not be predicted through a genetic test, which means that genetic tests do not offer the certainty they appear to provide.[89] Their conclusion that the campaign's "rhetorical characteristics of testimonials and language choices translate the technical and institutional complexity of genetic testing to the singular level of personal preference and control" is an incisive analysis of the Myriad campaign, and it also foregrounds a significant thread that pervades cancer prevention topoi more generally over the course of the twentieth century and into the present day, as individuals are encouraged to pursue control of their disease for the benefit of themselves and their families, but also as part of the public's demand for assurance that cancer can in fact be managed if only individuals do their part to address the risks.[90]

The volatile image of cancer prevention imposes multiple pressures on individuals charged with responsibility for fending off a disease whose unpredictability accounts for the urgent desire to be assured that correct action on the part of individuals will support the continued progress of society in spite of obstacles such as cancer. While access to the type of control promised in prevention topoi is never fully available to anyone, it is also important to recognize that even the limited control available through particular health measures is often embedded in a degree of privilege that is simultaneously invoked and suppressed in public arguments about cancer. To be sure, Epstein does acknowledge that higher cancer risks associated with race "are probably due to environmental factors rather than any intrinsic or genetic susceptibility," but his focus on prevention in a chapter titled "What You Can Do to Prevent Cancer" circles back to the themes of choice and agency in a way that elides the varying degrees with which certain populations are able to maintain the control he advocates.[91] While Epstein's extensive review of carcinogenic substances in that chapter makes available valuable insight into hazards individuals should be aware of, some of his conclusions overlook the material constraints that most people face in making career choices: "Unless you are fully and completely prepared to take the consequences, you should not go to work in an uncontrolled, high-risk industry, especially one with a bad track record."[92] He acknowledges that "if you are already working in one, you may have only very limited options, other than leaving," but his advice to those seeking work "to choose a large, well-organized plant with reliable and informed union-leadership, one in which carcinogens are handled in closed systems and the workplace is monitored with sensitive instrumentation" fails to acknowledge that many people do not have the luxury of shopping for working conditions that limit their exposure to carcinogens.[93] This line of argument simultaneously acknowledges the added danger of cancer created by industry and displaces the responsibility for its outcome on individuals who can simply choose not to work in those environments.

This tension continues to pervade environmental cancer activism in the present day. In analyzing the rhetorical strategies of Breast Cancer Action (BCA) and Breast Cancer Fund (BCF), two organizations founded in the 1990s by women whose personal experience had made them aware of the inadequacy of public information about breast cancer circulated through "pink ribbon culture," Karen Kopelson notes that both groups appeal "to uncertainty, fear, even chaos," but differently constitute audiences through the range of possible responses they make available.[94] Her nuanced article explores the strategies deployed on each organization's website in motivating people to act decisively to address the environmental concerns that play a role in the development of breast cancer. While she acknowledges BCF's success in constituting an audience that is persuaded to move beyond the "think pink" mainstream breast cancer culture, Kopelson notes that the website's emphasis on personal action to reduce environmental toxins in the home communicates the idea "that there are simple, nearly effortless things we can do—literally within arm's reach—to reduce our exposures to environmental hazards."[95] Although Kopelson notes that the BCA appeals to an already existing audience of believers in its persistent focus on breast cancer activism as a social justice initiative, she also makes the important point that the BCF's skill in inspiring people to think differently about breast cancer remains situated within "the relentless promotion of individualism in U.S. culture writ large," adding that "the class privilege assumed by these prevention tips and avoidance regimes is striking."[96] Like Epstein's newly enlightened employee whose agency includes simply refusing a job in which hazardous chemicals are used, the BCF's argument for social change circles back to a focus on the individual's control of the environment, predicated on the assumption that "individual women have nothing but money and time—to devote to protecting *the domestic sphere*."[97] In a similar vein, Emilia Nielsen notes that, while the environmental breast cancer movement casts "cancer risk as a collective concern," mainstream breast cancer culture's "emphasis on the learning of individual risk factors, knowing one's genetic predisposition, and early detection via regular mammograms can be framed to promote personal responsibility."[98] The project of Nielsen's *Disrupting Breast Cancer Narratives: Stories of Rage and Repair* includes highlighting the genre of disruptive narrative as a challenge to these mainstream discourses and the burden of responsibility that they impose on individuals with cancer.

PREVENTION AND THE LURE OF CONTROL

Although cancer prevention topoi have an important role in promoting public health, lines of argument that assert the potential to overcome cancer through strength of will, education, and intelligence have particular power in creating a people who are assured that cancer can be controlled and ultimately conquered at least in large measure through the actions of intelligent and informed individuals. As is the case with other cancer topoi, the promise of conquering cancer may not empower patients in the way people hope for but instead can implicitly constitute cancer patients as deficient, reinscribing what Sontag describes as the ancient view that disease comes from some flaw in character, "as forms of self-judgment, of self-betrayal."[99] Unfortunately, the interdependence between cancer prevention and access to certain types of personal choices, including a range of options pertaining to living space, work environments, and access to health care, reinforces a tendency in American society to assume that unlimited possibilities for autonomy exist, and that those who are able to achieve the promised control over their lives are those most willing to accept personal responsibility for their health. Although Emily Nye notes that cancer patients are more likely to be treated sympathetically than people who have AIDS, a careful look at the nuances of dominant cancer topoi suggests that representations of cancer may not entirely support Michael Bronski's interpretation that "cancer victims are usually 'innocent.'"[100] The persistence of these lines of argument despite ample evidence that reveals their limitations can be accounted for by recognizing the multiple ways in which the public's anxiety about cancer can be assuaged by even the most flawed promise that cancer can be controlled. As is true of the cancer topoi of war and positivity, the topos of cancer prevention imposes on enlightened individuals the responsibility for overcoming the damaging effects of civilization, ensuring that the promises of modern progress can be sustained even in the face of evidence that challenges the eugenic assumption that social well-being can be promoted through absolute faith in science, industry, and civilization.

5

Eugenic Reverberations

WHAT RHETORIC TELLS US ABOUT CANCER—AND OURSELVES

Cancer rhetorics provide only one example of an impulse to turn away from full engagement with problems in public health. Many people expressed bafflement over a similar phenomenon in the US response to the COVID-19 pandemic. Certainly, other countries struggled to devise effective responses to a novel, unpredictable, and lethal disease. However, the determination of US leaders to distance themselves entirely from the threat to public health posed by the spread of the virus was particularly surprising. The most notable evidence of this attempt came in former president Trump's repeated claim that the virus would just go away, which according to the *Washington Post* he had uttered nineteen times by July 2, 2020.[1] According to Trump, the later revelation that he in fact deliberately downplayed the effects of a virus that he knew to be deadly was based in his effort to "avoid panic." Commentators such as Tamara Keith have made note of a contradiction in Trump's willingness to incite panic in other areas, which underscores the former president's perception that issues pertaining to public health illustrate a type of vulnerability that uniquely jeopardized the image of national power he tried to maintain throughout his time in office.[2]

The former president's refusal to take responsibility for this pressing national problem can be seen as a distinctive feature of the complex political environment in the spring and summer of 2020. At the same time, it would be a mistake to assume that the strategy of wishing away public health problems came out of nowhere. Many people lamented Trump's refusal to issue a national mandate for preventive measures such as social distancing or wearing a mask in public, but it is also clear that this response resonated with many Americans. After all, many governors and local officials were eager to carry on the fight against vaccine and mask mandates long after Trump's departure from office, an approach supported by a large percentage of their constituents. While many people have considered these responses part of an unusually troubling political moment, history provides many examples of how the American conviction that anyone can thrive and flourish has been accompanied by the assumption that weakness is a choice that can and should be overcome, or at least should be set aside in the interests of those who embody the American ideal of power and resiliency. It is also based in the tendency to define the public good not according to measures that support vulnerable individuals, but according to standards of productivity and economic growth that are assumed to benefit everyone equally. In fact, the US emphasis on individualism always exists in tension with the pursuit of bringing people together in support of a collective good. This tension poses a notable challenge for rhetorics that engage with public health concerns.

The challenge of negotiating issues pertaining to public health is particularly evident as widely diverging views of the relationship between individual interests and the public good emerged during the pandemic. Although the scramble among medical researchers to understand COVID-19 has created confusion at times, it has been consistently clear that the disease poses a particular threat to the elderly and people with chronic medical conditions. In light of this fact, those who assume that the public good resides in economic security often cast their response to the pandemic in terms that simply removed the elderly and infirm from public life. According to this view, to inconvenience a population that has a limited role in the national economy is a small price to pay when weighed against what is seen as the ultimate social good of a thriving economy and consistent display of national strength. This assumption appeared to inform the response of Florida governor Ron DeSantis, who achieved notoriety early in the pandemic for his resistance to broad statewide measures to curb the coronavirus. Instead, Governor DeSantis issued orders for senior citizens and people with chronic illnesses to stay at home to protect themselves from exposure, a measure that in some respects located the responsibility for managing a public health crisis in the bodies of those individuals who were presumably most affected.[3] Although there are in fact alternatives to conceiving of economic prosperity and public health as opposing goals that require the choice of one or the other, the fact that the two have often been positioned in opposition to each other might be accounted for by the frequent assumption that there is no need to worry too much about the concerns of those who are not in the mainstream of social progress, profit, and production.

Although this book is explicitly about cancer rhetoric, my argument that representations of cancer are deeply embedded in cultural assumptions about who "we" are is relevant to other public health concerns, as well. Cancer rhetorics provide a particularly ubiquitous example of how the American emphasis on self-sufficiency and scientific progress has the potential to interfere with the ability of people who are sick and disabled to be seen. Confidence and self-sufficiency may be worthy American ideals, but when imposed on other people these qualities serve as weapons that allow those who are strong and fit to go about their business with the expectation that those who are vulnerable can (and should) rally and find their way back to "normal" life or suppress any evidence that this is not possible. Although eugenic ideologies do not have the widespread respectability that they had in the 1920s and 1930s, the pressure to overcome the ravaging effects of cancer, as well as other diseases and disabilities, through dispositions such as courage, a positive outlook, determination, and intelligence, reflects the entrenched presence of eugenic hopes for a modern society progressing toward strength and productivity untroubled by disabling conditions and poor health.

In his 1909 *Chapters in Eugenics*, Francis Galton wrote, "The first and main point is to secure the general intellectual acceptance of Eugenics as a hopeful and most important study. Then let its principles work into the heart of the nation, who will gradually give practical effect to them in ways that we may not wholly foresee."[4] This book has argued that persistent representations of cancer in the twentieth century derive from the "general intellectual acceptance of Eugenics," demonstrating how eugenic principles have shaped American views of health, chronic illness, and disability "in ways that we may not wholly foresee." While cancer research and clinical practice have led to remarkable gains in prognosis and treatment, the pace of medical progress has not been rapid enough to satisfy a public anxious to maintain confidence in American strength, ingenuity, and productivity. Across decades of the twentieth century, central topoi have both informed the public about current developments in cancer research and rhetorically constructed a people equipped for the intelligent, courageous, and forward-thinking response needed to sustain national progress.

This rhetorical approach emerges from the tension created when the explicit goal of making cancer visible comes up against the strong cultural impulse to suppress the harsh reality that such visibility brings to light. The opposition between the desire to see and not to see is also present in the history of disability. Sharon Snyder and David Mitchell describe the shift that takes place from premodern periods when the conception of disability "as a private family matter functioned as a form of social invisibility" to the nineteenth century, when the public visibility of disability forced people to account for disability as part of the life of the community.[5] Although cancer and other chronic illnesses differ from disability in key ways, there are important connections in the cultural function of bringing into view the uncomfortable specter of "the abnormal." As Rosemarie Garland-Thomson explains, "The category of disability exists as a way to exclude the kinds of bodily forms, functions, impairments, changes, or ambiguities that call into question our cultural fantasy of the body as a neutral, compliant, and predictable instrument of some transcendent will."[6] Cancer rhetoric's purpose is to make people aware of the need for early detection and prevention, but doing so also draws attention to a threat that must be suppressed by virtue of being made visible, a rhetorical endeavor that entails restoring a vision of the body as "a neutral, compliant, and predictable instrument." A rhetorical history of cancer must take material conditions into account, but it also acknowledges language as shaping material reality in ways that extend beyond the boundaries of medical protocols or the physical effects of disease.

A "kairotic account of medical history" illustrates the complexity that surrounds every interaction involving rhetoric and the body.[7] Jay Dolmage notes that "wherever we find the body rhetorically contested, and wherever we find rhetorical contestation about the body's role in meaning-making, we see intensely fraught negotiations."[8] To bring rhetoric into the history of cancer means acknowledging cancer as an embodied experience, which inevitably confronts the perpetual challenge of navigating a world that strives for perfection that bodies simply cannot attain. Dolmage's discussion of the implications that come from linking rhetoric and embodiment captures much of the complexity that surrounds dominant themes in twentieth-century cancer topoi: "Rhetoric is always embodied. When I say this, I mean, first, that all meaning issues forth from the body and that second, communication reaches into the body to shape its possibilities. The body has traditionally been both a rhetorical instrument and a rhetorical experiment, even as bodies have always been insistently material. The corpus of history has most often been shaped to look like an ideal body: proportional, autonomous, never needing the assistance of others, strong—and of course white and masculine and upright and forward-facing. But if you find the *rhetorical* body, you find a field of tension, a site of trial and trouble; find the body in history and you need rhetoric not just to uncover layers of evidence but also the negotiation, argument, and translation between them."[9] This project reflects the aim of "finding the body in history," as it has entailed using rhetoric as a lens for understanding cancer as not only a medical condition but also a cultural preoccupation with strength, control, and the performance of a body that comes into being through language about cancer—and that is consistently fraught with the "field of tension" that comes from a disease that at times resists even the most courageous, cheerful, and conscientious efforts possible.

The greatest threat coming from cancer is of course to human life itself. A secondary cultural concern comes from the inability of cancer patients to live up to what Iris Marion Young refers to as "the norm of the 'hale and hearty' worker."[10] As Lennard Davis notes, "Disabilities would be most dysfunctional in postindustrial countries, where the ability to perambulate or manipulate is so concretely tied to productivity, which in itself is tied to production."[11] The fact that this understanding is embedded in the discourse that informs the formation of the American Society for the Control of Cancer is evident in Lakeman's explicit statement that the "social problem" of cancer entails the recognition that statistics are valuable in revealing "the terrific onslaught of cancer against men and women at the most useful period of life and at the age when the care and guidance of children and the discharge of business responsibilities make the mother and father most valuable to society."[12] This comment illustrates S. Lochlann Jain's observation that "American economies simply do not prioritize health. No particular logic demands that a population's general health *should* trump other national concerns."[13] Although neither Lakeman nor other ASCC leaders suggest that the only reason for being concerned about cancer is its effect on the productivity of the American worker, attunement to the ideologies that shape cancer rhetoric and the topoi that dictate appropriate responses to cancer requires an awareness of the implications surrounding repeated references to the detrimental effects of cancer on the economy.

Numerous commentators have noted the further complication that in recent years the early philanthropic focus of cancer publicity has been subsumed by consumer culture, what Mary DeShazer describes as "the 'pink kitsch' of the cancer marketplace."[14] Samantha King argues that the shift from "breast cancer politics to breast cancer charity" has ironically narrowed the scope of responsibility for cancer from the community to individual generosity: "Contemporary discourses, strategies and tools of generosity reflect and produce a remolded view of America as a conflict-free and integrated nation whose survival depends on personal acts of philanthropy mediated through—and within—consumer culture. By according responsibility for the health and welfare of individuals to personal generosity, we simultaneously deploy a constricted understanding of the economic, political, social, and cultural forces that converge to shape problems of health and welfare."[15] This shift to individual responsibility connects with the longstanding impulse not to see the range of cancer experiences. Kate Pickert's description of METAvivor, an advocacy group for metastatic breast cancer patients, depicts the organization as challenging previous decades in which "the needs of such women have been overshadowed by a pink ribbon culture focused on 'survivors.'"[16] Phaedra Pezzullo's exploration of resistance to National Breast Cancer Awareness Month includes attention to the dangers that come about as the success of specific advocacy groups creates a monolithic discourse that elides the complexity that surrounds an issue such as breast cancer: "Because opposition to NBCAM is rarely heard, the discourse promoted by NBCAM arguably has become institutionalized as hegemonic 'common sense' in the current approach to breast cancer in the U.S."[17] As Karen Kopelson aptly notes, "'breast cancer culture,' singular, does not exist, or at least has never been the pink monolith Ehrenreich describes, though that it appears so is of the utmost significance and is part of her point."[18] Gayle A. Sulik's *Pink Ribbon Blues: How Breast Cancer Culture Undermines Women's Health* offers a trenchant critique of the effects that have come about through the illusion of a singular "breast cancer culture" that has come about as a result of the success of the Komen Foundation, a fundraising organization that has played a significant role in making breast cancer more visible: "Pink ribbon culture in the United States has become more than a cultural trend or a successful industry; it has become a distinct cultural system that is integrated into the fabric of American life. Grounded in advocacy, deeply held beliefs about gender and femininity, mass-mediated consumption, and the cancer industry, pink ribbon culture has transformed breast cancer from an important social problem that requires complicated social and medical solutions to a popular item for public consumption."[19]

Even as people with cancer face pressure to remain productive contributors to society, their disease has become a profitable industry that represents their cause in ways that further obscure their lived experiences. Cancer is so problematic because it attacks even the notion that one can attain the ideal body. The urgent imperative for cancer rhetoric is to reinscribe the viability of that image and the assumption that scientific progress is ongoing despite the disruptions represented by a disease that continues to have a pervasive presence even as there have been significant advances in cancer treatment. A historical perspective on cancer topoi demonstrates the complex factors that are at work as language about cancer becomes entwined with what Davis describes as a strong cultural impulse to normalize all experience: "Whether we are talking about AIDS, low-birth-weight babies, special education issues, euthanasia, and the thousand other topics listed in the newspaper every day, the examination, discussion, anatomizing of this form of difference is nothing less than people's desperate attempt to consolidate their normality."[20] As Jain suggests, such efforts ultimately impose pressure on people with cancer to devise practices that conceal their suffering to ensure that they don't make others uncomfortable, an approach that "turns cancer survivorship from an emotional and physical state into an ability, a private trait rather than a communal effort and responsibility."[21]

People with cancer experience the pressure "to consolidate their normality" in many different ways. In describing her visit from a representative from Reach for Recovery following her mastectomy, Audre Lorde focuses on her inability to overcome the gap that separated her from her visitor in spite of their shared experience with cancer: "I looked away, thinking, 'I wonder if there are any black lesbian feminists in Reach for Recovery?"[22] Lorde's awareness of her difference extended beyond the boundaries of identity to engage with her visitor's determination that she should normalize the effects of her disease, even to the extent of hiding them from herself: "Her message was, you are just as good as you were before because you can look exactly the same. Lambswool now, then a good prosthesis as soon as possible, and nobody'll ever know the difference. But what she said was, '*You'll* never know the difference,' and she lost me right there, because I knew sure as hell *I'd* know the difference."[23] Lorde's comment highlights the disjunction between the experiences of cancer patients who daily confront the abnormality of their situation and an environment in which the goal is to pretend that "you are just as good as you were before."

While rhetoric creates and perpetuates cultural attitudes, it can also promote awareness that might lead to alternative ways of communicating about the complex realities that surround us. Dolmage points out that rhetoric draws attention not only to the idealized images that have circumscribed bodies but "also [to] the negotiation, argument, and translation" needed to sift through historical evidence about people's lived experiences.[24] Although people with cancer may recognize the relevance of certain aspects of prominent cancer topoi, many patients have noted that dominant representations of cancer do not fully capture the reality of their experiences with illness. This gap can be addressed through cultivating rhetorical strategies that will offer alternatives to those focused on normality as the ultimate goal.

An important step in promoting such strategies will be the continued expansion of the range of participants in conversations about cancer. The rhetorical analysis in this book is primarily drawn from archival materials that reflect the discourse of the media, major cancer centers, and twentieth-century cancer activists and organizations. The book's primary analytical scope ends in the early 1990s, which constitutes a shift in cancer rhetoric that came about as "the politicized patient," coupled with an effective network of breast cancer activism, substantially expanded the range of participants who play an active role in language about cancer and medical policy.[25] In addition, the explosion of social media has provided cancer patients with new mechanisms for representing their own experiences. Although this book recognizes the importance of personal narratives in shaping cancer rhetoric in the early decades of the century, the technologies available since 1990, as well as social change that has encouraged wider representation of diverse points of view, have significantly increased the importance and scope of these narratives. Lorde summarized her disappointment in her encounter with the Reach for Recovery representative by writing, "I needed to talk with women who shared at least some of my major concerns and beliefs and visions, who shared at least some of my language."[26] Lorde, Sontag, and others committed to writing honestly about their experiences with cancer have provided a valuable foundation for others who have subsequently used writing as a way of expressing the range of their experiences with the disease and in the process have challenged the cultural emphasis on normalizing an experience that cannot be normal. These early writers have laid the groundwork for what Emilia Nielsen has documented as the "revitalization and proliferation" of breast cancer discourses through "disruptive cancer narratives" that "resist 'pink ribbon' culture with its primary focus on awareness and the promotion of early detection, cheerfulness, and adoption of the identity of 'survivor.'"[27]

At the same time, my goal in this book has been to resist any conception of history as functioning in a linear progression. My decision to end the analysis with the early 1990s and my acknowledgment that subsequent decades experience a substantial change in cancer rhetoric should not be interpreted as a sign that social media, cancer activism, and politicized patients offer a panacea for normalizing impulses found in cancer rhetorics of the past. The cultural pursuit of normalcy and self-sufficiency are too strong to imagine the disappearance of cancer topoi that urge the public to focus on the control of cancer and exhort cancer patients to agree that they'll "never know the difference."[28] A kairology of cancer rhetoric acknowledges that language has a powerful role in circulating resilient cultural ideologies that many people will find inadequate but will also find difficult to resist entirely.

If this book has a lesson, it is not that we can eliminate problematic rhetorical frameworks about cancer but that we can benefit from understanding the complexity of the language and images we use. The cancer topoi examined here are challenging not because they are problematic, but because they aren't entirely so. Even the war metaphor, which has been widely critiqued by many analysts and people with cancer, may facilitate reflection about the relationship between personal experience with disease and larger social and political concerns. Lorde strategically adopts the war metaphor following her diagnosis with breast cancer in order to interrogate the conditions in modern life that have enabled cancer to thrive: "Women with breast cancer are warriors, also. I have been to war, and still am."[29] Lorde's trenchant reflections capture the experience of many patients whose encounters with the resilience of the disease move them to conceive of themselves as soldiers fighting a sinister enemy whose tactics they can never fully anticipate—and whose causes may be embedded in the fabric of modern life in ways that have not yet been acknowledged.

Eli Clare describes this push and pull as present in every aspect of medical diagnosis: "Simply put, diagnosis wields immense power. It can provide us access to vital medical technology or shame us, reveal a path toward less pain or get us locked up. It opens doors and slams them shut."[30] Perhaps the best we can do is to immerse ourselves in the tensions we find in cancer rhetoric, in the process accepting the many nuances that any experience with illness brings. This entails resisting the impulse to rail against topoi that are an inevitable and even at times helpful element of human communication, but it also requires an awareness of the damaging implications particular metaphors might hold and a resistance to language that posits a monolithic medical subject or experience. Diedrich carefully considers the damage that comes from the fact that "sanctioned illness narratives dwell not on loss and failure but on *the overcoming of loss and failure*" (emphasis original); however, she stresses a response based on the insight that "there is not one, single, hegemonic counternarrative, but many."[31] Such an insight yields opportunities for transforming every term surrounding the cancer experience. Diedrich's analysis of the narrative of Eve Sedgwick includes the recognition that "shame is productive not only of normalizing identifications, but also of transgressive disidentifications"; for Sedgwick, the shame of illness can be seen as "creative of new ways of being and doing," a striking contrast to the externally imposed shame that isolated patients in the dark cancer wards of the nineteenth century.[32]

The next phase of cancer rhetoric will not be entirely free from the negative implications that are an inevitable part of the traditions that have pervaded cancer rhetoric across centuries. However, history suggests that these traditions can be productively informed by the infusion of the voices of those who have experienced cancer as a way of being that entails real suffering but also offers alternatives to the illusion of control that no one can attain and to eugenic orientations that should be banished from our social consciousness. In fact, Lorde argues that visibility for the cancer patient contains power in spite of, or perhaps because of, its uncontrollable nature: "That visibility which makes us most vulnerable is that which also is the source of our greatest strength."[33] Clare argues that the pursuit of a strong response to illness begins with living in the moment, for "if we choose to wait for the always-just-around-the-corner cures, lavishing them with resources, energy, and media attention, we risk suspending our present-day lives."[34] Such a response can be informed by Christa Teston's discussion of "dwelling," which "through the act not just of radical presence with but also radical response to disease and all its contributors, is one way of being attuned to and with a body in flux."[35] To pursue "radical presence" does not address all of the physical, mental, and emotional difficulties that cancer brings; nor does it conquer the problematic ideas embedded in dominant representations of cancer. However, attention to the rich and complex experiences of people with cancer, including a recognition of cancer as a force that is often difficult and disabling, may help to promote ways of experiencing and speaking about cancer that offer a deeper representation of its reality.

The pursuit of a deeper understanding of cancer begins with attention that does not immediately shift to normalizing the experience. Jain argues that "for cancer to be recognized as a scourge and as a violent visitation, it has to be acknowledged."[36] Truly acknowledging the complexity of cancer can offer care as a substitute for the careless expectation that people with cancer will respond to their disease in a manner that reassures everyone else that there's nothing to worry about. In offering care webs as a new social model, Leah Lakshmi Piepzna-Samarasinha asks, "What does it mean to shift our ideas of access and care (whether it's disability, childcare, economic access, or many more) from an individual chore, an unfortunate cost of having an unfortunate body, to a collective responsibility that's maybe even deeply joyful?"[37] According to Virginia Held, care ethics "promotes the values of building trust and mutual concern, and especially of responding to needs effectively, and with sensitivity and empathetic understanding."[38] Such an understanding opens the way for both people with cancer and those who care for them to counter the push for a norm that lacks the rich possibility available through a genuine encounter with the complexity of the full range of human experiences. A. Suresh Canagarajah describes this recognition as something he has achieved through confronting his own cancer diagnosis: "I don't want to leave readers with the impression that anomalous embodiment is only second best for all of us, or a form of consolation, in lieu of the ideal. Anomalous embodiment conveys that individual imperfections of many kinds are the stuff of life, and motivate attunement to social networks and environmental ecologies for anyone's ability."[39] He insists that this attunement leads to a new appreciation for collaborative relationships: "Disability justice should go beyond integrating the disabled into the market economy to reconfiguring the market and social structural conditions to accommodate people with diverse abilities in education and employment. These structural changes should also encourage inter-dependency among people as well as between people and the environment based on ethical values, beyond purely economic and market considerations."[40] Canagarajah's vision offers a useful counter to the eugenic emphasis on autonomy, strength, and progress that haunted cancer rhetorics across the twentieth century and that continues to be with us today.

The public response to the COVID pandemic shows that we are a long way from achieving this vision. In a 2020 *Vox* article Alice Wong describes the anxiety she has faced as an Asian American disabled person who regularly relies on a ventilator due to medical rationing during the pandemic, and she adds, "Eugenics isn't a relic from World War II, it's alive today, embedded in our culture, policies, and practices."[41] This book supports Wong's claim that eugenic ways of thinking are indeed "embedded in our culture, policies, and practices," but it doesn't have to be that way. Susan Wendell offers the provocative insight that chronic illness and disability offer "different *ways of being* that give valuable perspectives on life and the world."[42] For Wendell, these ways of being provide an important way of imagining the suffering illness brings that reflects neither a denial of reality nor fatalism: "If we could live the ways of being without the suffering, some of us would choose to live them. Some of us would choose to live them even if they were inseparable from the suffering. And some of us are glad to have been forced to live them, would choose to be rid of the suffering even if it meant losing the ways of being, but would hope to hold on to what we have learned from them."[43] To learn from suffering, to develop ways of being that embrace "anomalous embodiment," requires becoming aware of and resisting the subtle imposition of a cultural mandate to subsume suffering in a sunny vision of strength and normalcy that no individual or society can possibly attain. This requires a concerted effort to challenge value systems that have been with us for so long that we tend to take them for granted. Mounting such a challenge is hard work, as Jessica Restaino writes: "My sense is that interrogation and destabilization of this longing for control is essential, continuous work."[44] Engaging in the "essential, continuous work" of giving up on control entails recognizing the ways in which eugenics has become embedded in our world view "in ways that we may not wholly foresee."[45] This can be a first step in devising responses to illness and disability that reject the impulse of normativity and allow us to pursue "a different relationship to all our wanted and unwanted feelings as an ethical resource," an endeavor that can lead to a new way of being for the well and the unwell.[46]

NOTES

Introduction

1. Tom Crook, *Governing Systems: Modernity and the Making of Public Health in England, 1830–1910*, Berkeley Series in British Studies, vol. 11 (Oakland: University of California Press, 2016), 15.

2. Crook, *Governing Systems*, 15.

3. Crook, 15.

4. Michael McGee, "In Search of 'The People': A Rhetorical Alternative," *Quarterly Journal of Speech* 61, no. 3 (1975): 242.

5. McGee, "In Search," 243.

6. McGee, 243.

7. Sharon L. Snyder and David T. Mitchell, *Cultural Locations of Disability* (Chicago: University of Chicago Press, 2006), 46.

8. Cheryl Glenn, *Unspoken: A Rhetoric of Silence* (Carbondale: Southern Illinois University Press, 2004), 7.

9. Judy Z. Segal, *Health and the Rhetoric of Medicine* (Carbondale: Southern Illinois University Press, 2005), 75.

10. Snyder and Mitchell, *Cultural Locations of Disability*, 48–49.

11. Snyder and Mitchell, 48–49.

12. McGee, 242.

13. Susan Wendell, "Unhealthy Disabled: Treating Chronic Illnesses as Disabilities," in *The Disability Studies Reader*, ed. Lennard J. Davis (Mahwah, NJ: Routledge, 2013), 161.

14. Henri-Jacques Stiker, *A History of Disability*, trans. William Sayers (Ann Arbor: University of Michigan Press, 1999), 8.

15. Stiker, *History of Disability*, 8.

16. Annemarie Mol, *The Body Multiple: Ontology in Medical Practice* (Durham, NC: Duke University Press, 2003), 9.

17. Lynda Birke, "Bodies and Biology," in *Feminist Theory and the Body*, ed. Janet Price and Margrit Shildrick (New York: Routledge, 1999), 45.

18. A. Suresh Canagarajah, *Language Incompetence: Learning to Communicate through Cancer, Disability, and Anomalous Embodiment* (New York: Routledge, 2022), 5, E-book.

19. Rosemarie Garland-Thomson, *Extraordinary Bodies: Figuring Disability in American Culture and Literature* (New York: Columbia University Press, 1997), 8.

20. Kat Arney, "The Dark Connection between Cancer Research and the Eugenics Movement," podcast, Genetic Literacy Project: Science Not Ideology, online.

21. Qtd. in Allen M. Spiegel, "The Jeremiah Metzger Lecture: A Brief History of Eugenics in America: Implications for Medicine in the 21st Century," *Transactions of the American Clinical and Climatological Association* 130 (2019): 216–31, US National Library of Medicine/National Institutes of Health, online.

22. Susan Currell and Christina Cogdell, "Introduction," in *Popular Eugenics: National*

Efficiency and Mass Culture in the 1930s, ed. Susan Currell and Christina Cogdell (Athens: Ohio University Press, 2006), 6.

23. Jay Dolmage, *Academic Ableism: Disability and Higher Education* (Ann Arbor: University of Michigan Press, 2017), 11.

24. Dolmage, *Academic Ableism*, 11.

25. Snyder and Mitchell, 26.

26. Wendy Kline, "Eugenics in the United States," in *Oxford Handbook of the History of Eugenics*, ed. Alison Bashford and Philippa Levine (New York: Oxford University Press, 2010), 512.

27. Paul A. Lombardo, "Introduction: Looking Back at Eugenics," in *A Century of Eugenics in America: From the Indiana Experiment to the Human Genome Era*, ed. Paul A. Lombardo (Bloomington: Indiana University Press, 2011), 7.

28. Lombardo, "Introduction," 7.

29. Douglas C. Baynton, "Disability and the Justification of Inequality in American History," in *The New Disability History: American Perspectives*, ed. Paul K. Longmore and Lauri Umansky (New York: New York University Press, 2001), 35.

30. Baynton, "Disability and the Justification of Inequality," 35.

31. Baynton, 36.

32. Lombardo, 7.

33. Nirmala Erevelles, *Disability and Difference in Global Contexts: Enabling a Transformative Body Politic* (New York: Palgrave Macmillan, 2011), 29.

34. Iris Marion Young, quoted in Wendell, "Unhealthy Disabled," 168.

35. Henry Giroux, quoted in David T. Mitchell and Sharon L. Snyder, *The Biopolitics of Disability: Neoliberalism, Ablenationalism, and Peripheral Embodiment* (Ann Arbor: University of Michigan Press, 2015), 4.

36. Lennard J. Davis, *Enforcing Normalcy: Disability, Deafness, and the Body* (Brooklyn: Verso, 1995), 24.

37. Leah Ceccarelli, *On the Frontier of Science: An American Rhetoric of Exploration and Exploitation* (East Lansing: Michigan State University Press, 2013), 20.

38. Jackie Stacey, *Teratologies: A Cultural Study of Cancer* (Mahwah, NJ: Routledge, 1997), 240.

39. Brad Byrom, "A Pupil and a Patient: Hospital-Schools in Progressive America," in Longmore and Umansky, *New Disability History*, 135.

40. John Williams-Searle, "Cold Charity: Manhood, Brotherhood, and the Transformation of Disability," in Longmore and Umansky, 158.

41. K. Walter Hickel, "Medicine, Bureaucracy, and Social Welfare: The Politics of Disability Compensation for American Veterans of World War I," in Longmore and Umansky, 236, 238.

42. Elof Axel Carlson, "The Hoosier Connection: Compulsory Sterilization as Moral Hygiene," in Lombardo, *Century of Eugenics in America*, 11.

43. Carlson, "Hoosier Connection," 11.

44. Snyder and Mitchell, 49.

45. Carlson, 14.

46. Dolmage, *Academic Ableism*, 11.

47. McGee, 243.

48. Garland-Thomson, *Extraordinary Bodies*, 15.

49. Davis, *Enforcing Normalcy*, 149.

50. Rosemarie Garland-Thomson, "Seeing the Disabled: Visual Rhetorics of Popular

Photography," in Longmore and Umansky, 348.

51. Garland-Thomson, "Seeing the Disabled," 337.

52. Jay Dolmage, "Disability Rhetorics," in *The Cambridge Companion to Literature and Disability*, ed. Clare Barker and Stuart Murray (Cambridge, UK: Cambridge University Press, 2017), 215.

53. Mol, *Body Multiple*, 121.

54. Segal, *Health and the Rhetoric of Medicine*, 23.

55. Segal, 23.

56. Lisa Keränen, *Scientific Characters: Rhetoric, Politics, and Trust in Breast Cancer Research* (Tuscaloosa: University of Alabama Press, 2010), 22.

57. Christa Teston, *Bodies in Flux: Scientific Methods for Negotiating Uncertainty* (Chicago: University of Chicago Press, 2017), 77.

58. Siddhartha Mukherjee, *The Emperor of All Maladies: A Biography of Cancer* (New York: Scribner, 2010), 182.

59. Jay Dolmage, "The Circulation of Discourse through the Body," in "Octalog III: The Politics of Historiography in 2010," edited by Lois Agnew, Laurie Gries, and Zosha Stuckey, coauthored with Vicki Tolar Burton, Jay Dolmage, Jessica Enoch, Ronald L. Jackson II, LuMing Mao, Malea Powell, Arthur E. Walzer, Ralph Cintron, and Victor Vitanza, *Rhetoric Review* 30, no. 2 (2011): 114.

60. Curtis E. Lakeman, "Cancer as a Social Problem," lecture, National Conference of Charities and Correction, Memphis, Tennessee, May 15, 1913, Frederick L. Hoffman Papers, 1913–16, MS C 3 box 1 of 2, History of Medicine Division, National Library of Medicine.

61. Davis, 2.

62. Davis, 2.

63. Jay Timothy Dolmage, *Disability Rhetoric* (Syracuse, NY: Syracuse University Press, 2014), 141.

Chapter 1

1. Michael C. McGee, "In Search of 'The People': A Rhetorical Alternative," *Quarterly Journal of Speech* 61, no. 3 (1975): 243.

2. Walter Ross, *Crusade: The Official History of the American Cancer Society* (New York: Arbor House, 1987), 18.

3. Henri-Jacques Stiker, *A History of Disability*, trans. William Sayers (Ann Arbor: University of Michigan Press, 1999), 65.

4. Stiker, *History of Disability*, 159.

5. Stiker, 160.

6. Stiker, 160.

7. A. Suresh Canagarajah, *Language Incompetence: Learning to Communicate through Cancer, Disability, and Anomalous Embodiment* (New York: Routledge, 2022), 49, E-book.

8. Stiker, 160.

9. Charles P. Childe, *The Control of a Scourge, or How Cancer Is Curable* (New York: E. P. Dutton, 1907), vii.

10. Childe, *Control of a Scourge* 12, 9.

11. Childe, 13–14.

12. Curtis E. Lakeman, "Cancer as a Social Problem," lecture, National Conference of Charities and Correction, Memphis, Tennessee, May 15, 1913, Frederick L. Hoffman Papers, 1913–16, MS C 3 box 1 of 2, History of Medicine Division, National Library of Medicine.

13. American Society for the Control of Cancer, Statement of Purpose, 1913, Frederick L. Hoffman Papers, 1913–16, MS C 3 box 1 of 2, History of Medicine Division, National Library of Medicine.

14. Carolyn Miller, "The Presumptions of Expertise: The Role of Ethos in Risk Analysis," *Configurations* 11, no. 2 (2003): 185.

15. Frederick L. Hoffman, "The Statistical Evidence of the Increase in Cancer," Frederick L. Hoffman Papers, 1913–16, MS C 3 box 1 of 2, History of Medicine Division, National Library of Medicine.

16. Frederick L. Hoffman, letter to insurance company presidents, 1913, Frederick L. Hoffman Papers, 1913–16, MS C 3 box 1 of 2, History of Medicine Division, National Library of Medicine.

17. James T. Patterson, *The Dread Disease: Cancer and Modern American Culture* (Cambridge, MA: Harvard University Press, 1987), 75.

18. Ross, *Crusade*, 23.

19. Ross, 24.

20. S. Lochlann Jain, *Malignant: How Cancer Becomes Us* (Berkeley: University of California Press, 2013), 63.

21. Isaac F. Marcosson, "Cancer and Public Relations," 1943, American Society for the Control of Cancer, scrapbook 6 ("General Clippings, 1942–44), series 3, record group 375, Public Affairs Scrapbooks, Memorial Sloan Kettering Cancer Center Library and Archives (hereafter MSKCC), Rockefeller Archive Center (hereafter RAC).

22. "We Can't Cure Cancer by Shuddering!," *New York Herald Tribune*, February 15, 1946, scrapbook 8 ("Creation of Cancer Center, July 1945–March 1946), series 3, record group 375, Public Affairs Scrapbooks, MSKCC Library and Archives, RAC.

23. Kirsten E. Gardner, *Early Detection: Women, Cancer, and Awareness Campaigns in the Twentieth-Century United States* (Chapel Hill: University of North Carolina Press, 2006), 34.

24. Gardner, *Early Detection*, 34.

25. Diane B. Paul and James Moore, "The Darwinian Context: Evolution and Inheritance," in *The Oxford Handbook of the History of Eugenics*, ed. Alison Bashford and Philipa Levine (New York: Oxford University Press, 2010), 35.

26. Paul and Moore, "Darwinian Context," 35.

27. Robert W. Rydell, *World of Fairs: The Century-of-Progress Expositions* (Chicago: University of Chicago Press, 1993), 19.

28. Rydell, *World of Fairs*, 39.

29. Rydell, 106.

30. Rydell, 114–15.

31. Rydell, 40–41.

32. Rydell, 43.

33. Lauren Love, "U-M to Remove Little, Winchell Names from Campus Facilities, *University Record*, March 29, 2018 (University of Michigan); Liz Graves, "Auditorium Honoring Jackson Laboratory Founder C. C. Little to Be Renamed," *Mount Desert Islander*, September 20, 2021, online.

34. Clarence C. Little, "Cancer Can Be Cured," ca. 1940, reel 1, vol. 1 (1939–41), series 4, subseries 3, record group 375, Public Affairs Scrapbooks, MSKCC Library and Archives, RAC.

35. Little, "Cancer Can Be Cured."

36. Little.

37. Rydell, 43–44, 48.

38. Rydell, 48–49.
39. Rydell, 53.
40. Curtis E. Lakeman, "Introductory Remark," Public Meeting on the Control of Cancer, Portland, Oregon, June 18, 1915, Frederick L. Hoffman Papers, 1913–16, MS C 3 box 1 of 2, History of Medicine Division, National Library of Medicine.
41. Edward Reynolds, "Cancer a Controllable Disease: How the Women's Clubs Can Help the Less Intelligent," address at the Annual Meeting of the Massachusetts State Federation of Women's Clubs, Marion, IL, June 24, 1915, Frederick L. Hoffman Papers, 1913–16, MS C 3, box 2 of 2, National Library of Medicine.
42. Elof Axel Carlson, "The Hoosier Connection: Compulsory Sterilization as Moral Hygiene," in *A Century of Eugenics in America: From the Indiana Experiment to the Human Genome Era*, ed. Paul A. Lombardo (Bloomington: Indiana University Press, 2011), 21.
43. Carlson, "Hoosier Connection," 18–19.
44. Susan Currell, "Eugenic Decline and Recovery in Self-Improvement Literature of the Thirties," in *Popular Eugenics: National Efficiency and American Mass Culture in the 1930s*, ed. Susan Currell and Christina Cogdell (Athens: Ohio University Press, 2006), 45.
45. Currell, "Eugenic Decline," 46.
46. Jay Dolmage, *Academic Ableism* (Ann Arbor: University of Michigan Press, 2017), 16.
47. Currell, 47.
48. Currell, 48.
49. Currell, 48.
50. Currell, 52.
51. Currell, 52.
52. Rosemarie Garland-Thomson, "Seeing the Disabled: Visual Rhetorics of Popular Photography: Visual Rhetorics of Popular Photography," in *The New Disability History: American Perspectives*, ed. Paul K. Longmore and Lauri Umansky (New York: New York University Press, 2001), 337.
53. Lakeman, "Cancer as a Social Problem."
54. Garland-Thomson, "Seeing the Disabled," 348.
55. Alma Archer, "Read This and Shiver," *New York City Mirror*, December 19, 1945, scrapbook 7 (1945), series 4, subseries 3, record group 375, Public Affairs Scrapbooks, MSKCC Library and Archives, RAC.
56. Lennard Davis, *Enforcing Normalcy: Disability, Deafness, and the Body* (Brooklyn: Verso, 1995), 129.
57. Currell, 52.
58. Currell, 49.
59. Currell, 58.
60. "A Brave Story," *Trained Nurse and Hosp*, rev. Feb. 1940, reel 1, vol. 1 (1939–41), series 4, subseries 3, record group 375, Public Affairs Scrapbooks, MSKCC Library and Archives, RAC.
61. "History of Memorial Cancer Center," 1945, box 1 (1935–49), series 3, record group 375, Press Releases, MSKCC Library and Archives, RAC.
62. Mary Lasker, "Our Role in the Development of the American Cancer Society and Its Support for Research," 1955, Mary Lasker Papers, 1940–93, box 77 (1955), series 111: Topical Files, Columbia University Rare Book and Manuscript Library.
63. Siddhartha Mukherjee, *The Emperor of All Maladies: A Biography of Cancer* (New York: Scribner, 2010), 96.

64. Mukherjee, *Emperor of All Maladies*, 99.

65. Mukherjee, 115.

66. Simi Linton, "What Is Disability Studies?" *PMLA* 120, no. 2 (2005): 521.

67. Rosemarie Garland-Thomson, *Extraordinary Bodies: Figuring Physical Disability in American Culture and Literature* (New York: Columbia University Press, 1997), 15.

68. Mary Tobin, "This Street of Fear Ends in Hope and Help," *New York Post*, September 23, 1940, reel 1, vol. 1 (1939–41), series 4, subseries 3, record group 375, Public Affairs Scrapbooks, MSKCC Library and Archives, RAC.

69. Tasha Dubriwny, *The Vulnerable Empowered Woman: Feminism, Postfeminism, and Women's Health* (New Brunswick, NJ: Rutgers University Press, 2012), 2.

70. "Children's Cancer Real Challenge," *Elizabeth Daily Journal* (Elizabeth, NJ) reel 1, scrapbook 8 (July 1945–March 1946), series 4, subseries 3, record group 375, Public Affairs Scrapbooks, MSKCC Library and Archives, RAC.

71. "Children's Cancer Real Challenge"; "3-Year-Old Cancer Victim Wonders When Docs Will Fix Leg and Bring It Back to Him," *Knoxville News-Sentinel* (Knoxville, TN), January 7, 1946; "They let Charlie Keep Thinking He'll Get His Leg Back—For They Know He Won't Live," *Memphis Press-Scimitar* (Memphis, TN), January 7, 1946; "Dying Rutherford Lad's Parents Support Cancer Center Drive," *Passaic Herald-News* (Passaic, NJ), January 7, 1946, scrapbook 8: "Creation of Cancer Center" (July 1945–March 1946), series 4, subseries 3, record group 375, Public Affairs Scrapbooks, MSKCC Library and Archives, RAC.

72. *Passaic Herald-News* (Passaic, NJ), January 7, 1946, reel 1, scrapbook 8 (July 1945–March 1946), series 4, subseries 3, record group 375, Public Affairs Scrapbooks, MSKCC Library and Archives, RAC.

73. Erving Goffman, *Stigma: Notes on the Management of Spoiled Identity* (Englewood Cliffs, NJ: Prentice-Hall, 1963), 121.

74. Jay Timothy Dolmage, *Disability Rhetoric* (Syracuse, NY: Syracuse University Press, 2014), 39.

75. Dolmage, *Disability Rhetoric*, 39–40.

76. Frank Horsfall, letter of protest to John Heller, n.d., folder 36, box 2 (1961–69), series 6, record group 375, TV/Radio, MSKCC Library and Archives, RAC.

77. Archer, "Read This and Shiver."

78. Davis, *Enforcing Normalcy*, 13.

79. Davis, 113.

80. Susan Sontag, *Illness as Metaphor and AIDS and Its Metaphors* (New York: Farrar, Straus and Giroux, 1977), 87.

Chapter 2

1. Ulrich Teucher, "The Therapeutic Psychopoetics of Cancer Metaphors: Challenges in Interdisciplinarity," *History of Intellectual Culture* 3, no. 1 (2003): 4.

2. Judy Z. Segal, "Public Discourse and Public Policy: Some Ways That Metaphor Constrains Health (Care)," *Journal of Medical Humanities* 18, no. 4 (1997): 219.

3. Jackie Stacey, *Teratologies: A Cultural Study of Cancer* (New York: Routledge, 1997), 63.

4. Teucher, "Therapeutic Psychopoetics," 1.

5. Susan Sontag, *Illness as Metaphor and AIDS and Its Metaphors* (New York: Farrar, Straus and Giroux, 1977), 3.

6. Sontag, *Illness as Metaphor*, 3.

7. Jeanne Fahnestock, *Rhetorical Figures in Science* (New York: Oxford University Press, 1999), 5.

8. Kenneth Burke, *Permanence and Change* (Berkeley: University of California Press, 1954), 95.

9. Stacey, *Teratologies*, 51.

10. Segal, "Public Discourse and Public Policy," 218.

11. Segal, "Public Discourse and Public Policy," 219.

12. Segal, "Public Discourse and Public Policy," 221; Teucher, 4.

13. Sonja K. Foss, *Rhetorical Criticism: Exploration and Practice*, 4th ed. (Long Grove, IL: Waveland, 2009), 97.

14. James T. Patterson, *The Dread Disease: Cancer and Modern American Culture* (Cambridge, MA: Harvard University Press, 1987), 31.

15. James S. Olson, *Making Cancer History: Disease and Discovery at the University of Texas M.D. Anderson Cancer Center* (Baltimore: Johns Hopkins University Press, 2009), 17.

16. Walter Ross, *Crusade: The Official History of the American Cancer Society* (New York: Arbor House, 1987), 30–31.

17. Patterson, *Dread Disease*, 31; "New Scientific Facts about Cancer," *New York Journal-American*, November 8, 1942, scrapbook 5.2 (January 1941–March 1942), series 4, subseries 3, record group 375, Public Affairs Scrapbooks, MSKCC Library and Archives, RAC.

18. Thanks to Adam Newman for sharing this insight in response to my presentation at the 2016 RSA Conference.

19. Eva-Maria Ziege, "Patterns within Prejudice: Antisemitism in the United States in the 1940s," *Patterns of Prejudice* 46, no. 2 (2012): 93–127.

20. Press release (Clarence Little announcement), folder 12, box 1, series 3, record group 375, Public Affairs Press Releases, MSKCC Library and Archives, RAC.

21. Press release (Harry Schoenfeld announcement), folder 12, box 1, series 3, record group 375, Public Affairs Press Releases, MSKCC Library and Archives, RAC.

22. "Elsa Maxwell's Party Line—An Offer of Hope," *New York Post*, December 5, 1945, scrapbook 6 (General Clippings, 1942–44), series 4, subseries 3, record group 375, Public Affairs Scrapbooks, MSKCC Library and Archives, RAC.

23. "Sloan Kettering Institute Opens Fight in Effort to Solve Cancer Source and Cure," *Dayton Daily News* (Dayton, OH), February 11, 1946, scrapbook 8 ("Creation of Cancer Center, July 1945–March 1946"), series 4, subseries 3, record group 375, Public Affairs Scrapbooks, MSKCC Library and Archives, RAC.

24. Curtis E. Lakeman, "Introductory Remarks," June 18, 1915, Public Meeting on the Control of Cancer, American Society for the Control of Cancer, Frederick L. Hoffman Papers, 1913–16, MS C 3 box 1 of 2, History of Medicine Division, National Library of Medicine.

25. "New Battleground in Cancer War," *New York Herald Tribune*, ca. 1940, reel 1, vol. 1 (1939–41), series 4, subseries 3, record group 375, Public Affairs Scrapbooks, MSKCC Library and Archives, RAC; George Britt, "Cancer Fight Gaining Elements of Success," *World Telegram*, 840, reel 1, vol. 1 (1939–41), series 4, subseries 3, record group 375, Public Affairs Scrapbooks, MSKCC Library and Archives, RAC.

26. "Power in Ingenuity: Lehigh President Addresses Patent Lawyers' Dinner," *New York Sun*, March 8, 1940, reel 1, vol. 1 (1939–41), series 4, subseries 3, record group 375, Public Affairs Scrapbooks, MSKCC Library and Archives, RAC.

27. "The Counterattack on Cancer," *New York World-Telegram*, January 18, 1946, scrapbook 9 (1946), series 4, subseries 3, record group 375, Public Affairs Scrapbooks, MSKCC Library and Archives, RAC.

28. Daniel Sarewitz, "Saving Science," *New Atlantis: A Journal of Technology and Society*, Spring/Summer 2016, online.

29. George Annas, "Reframing the Debate on Health Care: Reform by Replacing Our Metaphors," *New England Journal of Medicine* 332, no. 11 (1995): 745.

30. James S. Olson, *Bathsheba's Breast: Women, Cancer, and History* (Baltimore: Johns Hopkins University Press, 2002), 74–75.

31. "Chemical Warfare Officers Honored," *New York Journal-American*, May 6, 1945, scrapbook 5.2 (January 1941–March 1942), series 4, subseries 3, record group 375, Public Affairs Scrapbooks, MSKCC Library and Archives, RAC.

32. Siddhartha Mukherjee, *The Emperor of All Maladies: A Biography of Cancer* (New York: Scribner, 2010), 92.

33. "Cancer-Fighter Cornelius P. Rhoads: 'Some Gangsters Are Vulnerable,'" *Time*, June 27, 1949, online.

34. "New Cancer Hospital to Be Dedicated Tomorrow: X-Ray Machine with Power of $90,000,000 Worth of Radium to Push Battle," *New York Post*, June 13, 1939, scrapbook 2 (Hospital Opening, 1939), series 4, subseries 3, record group 375, Public Affairs Scrapbooks, MSKCC Library and Archives, RAC.

35. "Dispatch from the Front," *Hospital Topics and Buyer (Chicago)*, July 1, 1939, scrapbook 3: Hospital Opening (June 1939–December 1939), series 4, subseries 3, record group 375, Public Affairs Scrapbooks, MSKCC Library and Archives, RAC.

36. "Memorial Clinic Opens Tomorrow with Every Modern Weapon in War on Death," *New York Journal American*, June 18, 1939, scrapbook 2 (Hospital Opening 1939), series 4, subseries 3, record group 375, Public Affairs Scrapbooks, MSKCC Library and Archives, RAC; "New Hospital Wages Modern War on Cancer," *Fresno Bee-Republic*, June18, 1939, scrapbook 3: Hospital Opening (June 1939–December 1939), series 4, subseries 3, record group 375, MSKCC Library and Archives, RAC; "Radium Moved across Town: Four Grams Transferred to New Cancer Hospital—Shipment Worth $100,000, Bomblike Leaden Container Is Guarded by Police," *New York Sun*, June 23, 1939, scrapbook 3: Hospital Opening (June 1939–December 1939), series 4, subseries 3, record group 375, MSKCC Library and Archives, RAC.

37. "By Other Editors," *Savannah Morning News* (GA), July 26, 1942, also printed in the *New York Telegram* and as "The War on Cancer" in the *Grand Junction Daily Sentinel* (Grand Junction, CO), July 27, 1942, scrapbook 6: General Clippings (1942–44), series 4, subseries 3, record group 375, Public Affairs Scrapbooks, MSKCC Library and Archives, RAC.

38. Robert D. Potter, "Latest News about Cancer," *American Weekly* 1943, scrapbook 6: General Clippings (1942–44), series 4, subseries 3, record group 375, Public Affairs Scrapbooks, MSKCC Library and Archives, RAC.

39. Hon. Jacob Gould Schurman, address at the dedication of Memorial Hospital, June 14, 1939. box 1 (1935–49), series 3, record group 375, Press Releases, MSKCC Library and Archives, RAC.

40. New York Cancer Institute Social Service Auxiliary Brochure, 1944, Mary Lasker Papers, 1940–1993, box 75, series 111: Topical Files, Columbia University Rare Book and Manuscript Collection.

41. Olson, *Making Cancer History*, 54.

42. "Cancer and the Public," Memorial Hospital press release, May 14, 1944, folder 10, box 1 (1935–49), series 3, record group 375, Press Releases, MSKCC Library and Archives, RAC.

43. "Mustard Gas Offered to Fight Blood Cancer," *Geneva Times* (Geneva, NY), April 9, 1946, scrapbook 6: General Clippings (1942–44), series 4, subseries 3, Public Affairs Scrapbooks, MSKCC Library and Archives, RAC.

44. "Kettering Foundation Laboring on Substance to Trace Cancer—Scientists Study

Addition of Radioactive Atom to Test Solution Causing Disease," *Atlanta Journal*, September 29, 1946, scrapbook 6: General Clippings (1942–44), series 4, subseries 3, record group 375, Public Affairs Scrapbooks, MSKCC Library and Archives, RAC.

45. *New York Journal of Commerce*, December 12, 1946, scrapbook 8: "Creation of Cancer Center"(July 1945–March 1946), series 4, subseries 3, Public Affairs Scrapbooks, MSKCC Library and Archives, RAC.

46. "Williams Cites Invention, Not Battle, as Vital: Lehigh's President Stresses Role of Science in Talk to NY Patent Lawyers," reel 1, vol. 1 (1939–41), series 4, subseries 3, Public Affairs Scrapbooks, MSKCC Library and Archives, RAC.

47. Edwin B. Wilson, letter to Mary Lasker, June 18, 1953, Mary Lasker Papers, 1940–93, box 76, series 111: Topical Files, Columbia University Rare Book and Manuscript Collection.

48. "Sloan, Kettering to Combat Cancer—Former Makes a $4,000,000 Grant for Research Institute to Be Directed by the Latter," *New York Times*, August 8, 1945, scrapbook 6: General Clippings (1942–44), series 4, subseries 3, record group 375, MSKCC Library and Archives, RAC.

49. "Sloan, Kettering to Combat Cancer."

50. Oscar Ewing, "Address," April 16, 1948, folder 14, box 1, series 3, record group 375, Public Affairs Scrapbooks, MSKCC Library and Archives, RAC.

51. Paul C. Aebersold, "Atomic Developments and Technology in Cancer Research," talk given at Panel Discussion on "Participation in Medical Research by Technology," at the opening of the Sloan-Kettering Institute for Cancer Research, New York City, April 16, 1948, folder 14, box 1, series 3, record group 375, Public Affairs Files, MSKCC Library and Archives, RAC.

52. "Industry Tackles Cancer," *New York Sun*, August 11, 1945, scrapbook 6: General Clippings (1942–44), series 4, subseries 3, record group 375, Public Affairs Scrapbooks, MSKCC Library and Archives, RAC.

53. "Organized Cancer Research," *Santa Barbara News-Press* (Santa Barbara, CA), August 29, 1945, scrapbook 6: General Clippings (1942–44), series 4, subseries 3, record group 375, Public Affairs Scrapbooks, MSKCC Library and Archives, RAC.

54. "Lay Mind Has Confused Idea of Cancer Research," *Monticello Evening News* (Monticello, NY), December 15, 1945, scrapbook 7 (1945), series 4, subseries 3, record group 375, Public Affairs Scrapbooks, MSKCC Library and Archives, RAC.

55. Aebersold, "Atomic Developments and Technology in Cancer Research," 3.

56. "Both Destructive and Conservative," *Phoenix Republic* (Phoenix, AZ), August 19, 1945, scrapbook 6: General Clippings (1942–44), series 4, subseries 3, record group 375, Public Affairs Scrapbooks, MSKCC Library and Archives, RAC.

57. "Research for Life and Death," *San Francisco News*, September 3, 1945, scrapbook 6: General Clippings (1942–44), series 4, subseries 3, record group 375, Public Affairs Scrapbooks, MSKCC Library and Archives, RAC.

58. "Dr. Daniel A. Poling, Americans All," *Stamford Advocate* (Stamford, CT), September 1, 1945, scrapbook 6: General Clippings (1942–44), series 4, subseries 3, record group 375, Public Affairs Scrapbooks, MSKCC Library and Archives, RAC.

59. "One-Minute Spot Announcement: Series C, no. 3"; "One-Minute Spot Announcement: Series C, no. 2," Memorial Cancer Center Fund, folder 11, box 1, series 3, record group 375, Public Affairs Scrapbooks, MSKCC Library and Archives, RAC.

60. Edmund E. Day, "Memorial Cancer Center—A Commanding Cause," December 13, 1949, folder 15, box 1, series 3, record group 375, Public Affairs Scrapbooks, MSKCC Library and Archives, RAC.

61. *New York Times*, January 21, 1944, scrapbook 6: General Clippings (1942–44), series 4, subseries 3, record group 375, Public Affairs Scrapbooks, MSKCC Library and Archives, RAC.

62. Fuller Warren, "Facts and Figures by Fuller Warren," February 6, 1948, Mary Lasker Papers, 1940–93, folder 8 (1948), box 75, series 111: Topical Files, Columbia University Rare Book and Manuscript Collection.

63. Albert Rosenfeld, "A Superplan to Cut Years Off the War," *Life*, November 18, 1966, p. 108, Mary Lasker Papers, 1940–93, box 79, series 111: Topical Files, Columbia University Rare Book and Manuscript Library.

64. American Cancer Society, "Aiming Magic Bullets at Cancer," 1956 brochure, Mary Lasker Papers, 1940–93, box 77, series 111: Topical Files, Columbia University Rare Book and Manuscript Collection.

65. Olson, *Making Cancer History*, 231.

66. "Ask Ann Landers," *Richmond Times-Dispatch*, October 10, 1971, Mary Lasker Papers, 1940–93, box 79, series 111: Topical Files, Columbia University Rare Book and Manuscript Collection.

67. *Washington Post*, August 1, 1973, Mary Lasker Papers, 1940–93, box 80 ("Cancer 1973"), series 111: Topical Files, Columbia University Rare Book and Manuscript Collection.

68. "Cancer's Sniper War: Some Scientists Say Anticancer Spending Is Unwise, Retards Other Medical Research," *National Observer*, week ending July 20, 1974, Mary Lasker Papers, 1940–93, box 80 ("Cancer June 1974"), series 111: Topical Files, Columbia University Rare Book and Manuscript Library.

69. Judy Z. Segal, "Breast Cancer Narratives as Public Rhetoric: Genre Itself and the Maintenance of Ignorance," *Linguistics and the Human Sciences* 3, no. 1 (2007): 4.

70. Azra Raza, *The First Cell and the Human Costs of Pursuing Cancer to the Last* (New York: Hachette Book Group, 2019), 208.

71. Kristen Lindgren, "Bodies in Trouble: Identity, Embodiment, and Disability," in *Gendering Disability*, edited by Bonnie G. Smith and Beth Hutchison (New Jersey: Rutgers University Press, 2004), 154.

72. Lindgren, "Bodies in Trouble," 154, 155; Sontag, 84.

73. Henri-Jacques Stiker, *A History of Disability*, trans. William Sayers (Ann Arbor: University of Michigan Press, 1999), 8.

74. "A Child's Death Spurs the War against Cancer," *New York Herald Tribune*, February 7, 1946; "Boy's Death Spurs Fight on Cancer," *New York Times*, February 7, 1946, scrapbook 8: Creation of Cancer Center (July 1945–March 1946), series 4, subseries 3, record group 375, Public Affairs Scrapbooks, MSKCC Library and Archives, RAC.

75. "Heroic Lad of 3 Dies of Cancer," *New York Journal-American*, February 6, 1946, scrapbook 8: Creation of Cancer Center (July 1945–March 1946), series 4, subseries 3, record group 375, Public Affairs Scrapbooks, MSKCC Library and Archives, RAC.

76. Segal, "Breast Cancer Narratives as Public Rhetoric," 5.

77. Sontag, 64.

78. Sontag, 57.

79. A. Suresh Canagarajah, *Language Incompetence: Learning to Communicate through Cancer, Disability, and Anomalous Embodiment* (New York: Routledge, 2022), 4–5, E-book.

80. Susan Currell, "Eugenic Decline and Recovery in Self-Improvement Literature of the Thirties," in *Popular Eugenics: National Efficiency and American Mass Culture in the 1930s*, ed. Susan Currell and Christina Cogdell (Athens: Ohio University Press, 2006), 46.

81. Currell, "Eugenic Decline," 47.

82. Stacey, 44.

83. Stacey, 240.

84. Kristen Garrison, "The Personal Is Rhetorical: War, Protest, and Peace in Breast Cancer Narratives," *Disability Studies Quarterly* 27, no. 4 (2007).

85. Segal, "Public Discourse and Public Policy," 223.

86. Christa Teston, *Bodies in Flux: Scientific Methods for Mapping Medical Uncertainty* (Chicago: University of Chicago Press, 2017), 55.

87. Stacey, 62; Segal, "Public Discourse and Public Policy," 224.

88. Teucher, 4.

89. Segal, "Public Discourse and Public Policy," 228.

Chapter 3

1. Barbara Ehrenreich, *Bright-Sided: How the Relentless Promotion of Positive Thinking Has Undermined America* (New York: Metropolitan Books, 2009), 40, 42.

2. Ehrenreich, *Bright-Sided*, 41.

3. Ehrenreich, 41–42.

4. Audre Lorde, *The Cancer Journals, Special Edition* (1980; repr. San Francisco: Aunt Lute Books, 1997), 76.

5. Sharon L. Snyder and David T. Mitchell, *Cultural Locations of Disability* (Chicago: University of Chicago Press, 2006), 46.

6. Snyder and Mitchell, *Cultural Locations of Disability*, 47; Lorde, *Cancer Journals*, 76.

7. Susan Currell, "Eugenic Decline and Recovery in Self-Improvement Literature of the Thirties," in *Popular Eugenics: National Efficiency and American Mass Culture in the 1930s*, ed. Susan Currell and Christina Cogdell (Athens: Ohio University Press, 2006), 47.

8. Sara Ahmed, *The Promise of Happiness* (Durham, NC: Duke University Press, 2010), 59.

9. Currell, "Eugenic Decline," 48.

10. Siddhartha Mukherjee, *The Emperor of All Maladies: A Biography of Cancer* (New York: Scribner, 2010), 48.

11. Mukherjee, *Emperor of All Maladies*, 49; James S. Olson, *Making Cancer History: Disease and Discovery at the University of Texas M.D. Anderson Cancer Center* (Baltimore: Johns Hopkins University Press, 2009), 71.

12. James S. Olson, *Bathsheba's Breast: Women, Cancer, and History* (Baltimore: Johns Hopkins University Press, 2002), 158–59.

13. Olson, *Bathsheba's Breast*, 159.

14. "A Cheerful Institution," *West of Central Park*, 1935, folders 1–15, box 1 (1935–49), series 3, record group 375, Press Releases, MSKCC Library and Archives, RAC.

15. "Getting Ready for Christmas," *New York Herald Tribune*, December 20, 1939, scrapbook 4 (October 1939–December 1939), series 4, subseries 3, record group 375, Public Affairs Scrapbooks, MSKCC Library and Archives, RAC.

16. Press release, September 25, 1951, box 2, series 3, record group 375, Press Releases (1950–57), MSKCC Library and Archives, RAC.

17. Press release, May 20, 1964, folder 39 (1964), box 3, series 3, record group 375, Press Releases, MSKCC Library and Archives, RAC.

18. Caroline Keller, "Raising the Cancer Patient's Morale," *American Journal of Nursing* 49, no. 8 (1949), folder 16 (1950), box 2, series 3, record group 375, Press Releases (1950–57), MSKCC Library and Archives, RAC.

19. Memorial Center Report, December 1951, folder 17, box 2, series 3, record group 375, Press Releases (1950–57), MSKCC Library and Archives, RAC.

20. Michael Braun, "Classics in Oncology: Portrait of Arthur M. Sutherland, MD," *CA-A Cancer Journal for Clinicians* 31, no. 3 (May/June 1981), 157.

21. Qtd. in "'Psychological Invalidism' a Danger to Cancer Patients," 1954, Press Release to Science Writers, folder 20, box 2, series 3, record group 375, Press Releases, MSKCC Library and Archives, RAC.

22. Press release, February 23, 1960, folder 2, box 3, series 3, record group 375, Press Releases, MSKCC Library and Archives, RAC.

23. Press release, February 23, 1960, folder 2, box 3, series 3, record group 375, Press Releases, MSKCC Library and Archives, RAC.

24. Press release, October 26, 1977, folder 25, box 3, series 3, record group 375, Press Releases, MSKCC Library and Archives, RAC.

25. Press release, May 18, 1978, folder 44, box 5, series 3, record group 375, Press Releases, MSKCC Library and Archives, RAC.

26. Press release, May 14, 1979, folder 45 (1979), box 5, series 3, record group 375, Press Releases, MSKCC Library and Archives, RAC.

27. MD Anderson Annual Reports, 1950–51, Historical Resources Center, Research Medical Library, University of Texas MD Anderson Cancer Center.

28. MD Anderson Annual Reports, 1950–51.

29. Press release, October 14, 1968, folder 34, box 4, series 3, record group 375, Press Releases, MSKCC Library and Archives, RAC.

30. Press release, April 9, 1951, box 2, series 3, Press Releases (1950–57), record group 375, MSKCC Library and Archives, RAC.

31. Press release, April 9, 1951, box 2, series 3, Press Releases (1950–57), record group 375, MSKCC Library and Archives, RAC.

32. Press release, March 1966, folder 32, box 4, series 3, record group 375, Press Releases, MSKCC Library and Archives, RAC.

33. MD Anderson Annual Reports, 1951–52, Historical Resources Center, Research Medical Library, University of Texas MD Anderson Cancer Center.

34. MD Anderson Annual Reports, 1952–53, Historical Resources Center, Research Medical Library, University of Texas MD Anderson Cancer Center.

35. MD Anderson Annual Reports, 1954–55, Historical Resources Center, Research Medical Library, University of Texas MD Anderson Cancer Center.

36. MD Anderson Annual Reports, 1959–60, Historical Resources Center, Research Medical Library, University of Texas MD Anderson Cancer Center.

37. MD Anderson Annual Reports, 1974–76, Historical Resources Center, Research Medical Library, University of Texas MD Anderson Cancer Center.

38. "Rehabilitation Can't Begin Too Soon," *Memorial Sloan-Kettering News*, April 3, 1978, folder 44, box 5, series 3, record group 375, Press Releases, MSKCC Library and Archives, RAC.

39. Julia Bowman, "Functional Living Means Talking," *Conquest* 2, no. 3 (Winter 1988), Historical Resources Center, Research Medical Library, University of Texas MD Anderson Cancer Center.

40. "Matching Desire and Potential," *Conquest* 2, no. 3 (Winter 1988), Historical Resources Center, Research Medical Library, University of Texas MD Anderson Cancer Center.

41. Frederick L. Hoffman, "The Control of Cancer" lecture outline, n.d. (ca. 1914?),

Frederick L. Hoffman Papers, 1913–16, MS C 3 box 1 of 2, History of Medicine Division, National Library of Medicine.

42. Frederick L. Hoffman, note on Cyrus L. Topliff's "The Cancer Problem," printed in *Scientific American*, 1916, Frederick L. Hoffman Papers, 1913–16, MS C 3 box 1 of 2, History of Medicine Division, National Library of Medicine.

43. Currell, 48.

44. Curtis E. Lakeman, "Cancer as a Social Problem," address to the National Conference of Charities and Correction, Memphis, TN, May 15, 1913, Frederick L. Hoffman Papers, 1913–16, MS C 3 Box 1 of 2, History of Medicine Division, National Library of Medicine.

45. *Conquest* 2, no. 3 (Winter 1988), Historical Resources Center, Research Medical Library, University of Texas MD Anderson Cancer Center.

46. "A Nurse's Brag Book," *Conquest* 2, no. 3 (Winter 1988), Historical Resources Center, Research Medical Library, University of Texas MD Anderson Cancer Center.

47. "Valiant Is the Word: Tooth Bests Dorothy: Weeps at Ache, Though She Smiled at Amputation," *New York Journal America*, October 11, 1939, scrapbook 4 (October 1939–December 1939), series 4, subseries 3, record group 375, Public Affairs Scrapbooks, MSKCC Library and Archives, RAC.

48. "Valiant Is the Word."

49. "Smiles at Trouble," *Shenandoah Herald* (Shenandoah, PA), October 11, 1939, scrapbook 4 (October 1939–December 1939), series 4, subseries 3, record group 375, Public Affairs Scrapbooks, MSKCC Library and Archives, RAC.

50. Rosemarie Garland-Thomson, *Extraordinary Bodies: Figuring Physical Disability in American Culture and Literature* (New York: Columbia University Press, 1997), 15.

51. Erving Goffman, *Stigma: Notes on the Management of Spoiled Identity* (Hoboken, NJ: Prentice-Hall, 1963), 122.

52. Olson, *Making Cancer History*, 73.

53. Olson, *Making Cancer History*, 74.

54. Lorde, *Cancer Journals*, 76; Snyder and Mitchell, 46.

55. S. Lochlann Jain, *Malignant: How Cancer Becomes Us* (Berkeley: University of California Press, 2013), 47.

56. Henri-Jacques Stiker, *A History of Disability*, trans. William Sayers (Ann Arbor: University of Michigan Press, 1999), 160.

57. Snyder and Mitchell, 47.

58. "Biography of a Cancer," CBS Reports transcript, April 21, 1960, folder 27, series 4, subseries 3, record group 375, MSKCC Library and Archives, RAC.

59. Ehrenreich, 26.

60. Stiker, *History of Disability*, 160.

61. Ehrenreich, 33.

62. Frederick L. Hoffman, note on Cyrus L. Topliff's "The Cancer Problem," printed in *Scientific American*, 1916; Curtis E. Lakeman, "Introductory Remark," Public Meeting on the Control of Cancer, Portland, Oregon, June 18, 1915, Frederick L. Hoffman Papers, 1913–16, MS C 3 box 1 of 2, History of Medicine Division, National Library of Medicine.

63. Louise Woodstock, "Think about It: The Misbegotten Promise of Positive Thinking Discourse," *Journal of Communication Inquiry* 31, no. 2 (2007): 270.

64. Woodstock, "Think about It," 176–77.

65. Woodstock, 177.

66. Currell, 52.

67. Richard I. Evans, *Dialogue with C. G. Jung*, Dialogues in Contemporary Psychology Series (New York: Praeger, 1981), 145–46.

68. Evans, *Dialogue with C. G. Jung*, 145.

69. Olson, *Bathsheba's Breast*, 160.

70. Olson, *Making Cancer History*, 87–88.

71. Lawrence LeShan, *You Can Fight for Your Life: Emotional Factors in the Treatment of Cancer* (New York: M. Evans, 1977), 91, 2.

72. LeShan, *You Can Fight*, 18.

73. LeShan, 32–34.

74. LeShan, 34, 39.

75. LeShan, 117.

76. Carl O. Simonton, Stephanie Matthew-Simonton, and James Creighton, *Getting Well Again: A Step-by-Step, Self-Help Guide to Overcoming Cancer for Patients and Their Families* (New York: J. P. Tarcher, 1978), 3.

77. Simonton, Matthew-Simonton, and Creighton, *Getting Well Again*, 4, 5.

78. Simonton, Matthew-Simonton, and Creighton, 5.

79. Simonton, Matthew-Simonton, and Creighton, 9.

80. Simonton, Matthew-Simonton, and Creighton, 3, 26.

81. Simonton, Matthew-Simonton, and Creighton, 10, 11.

82. Simonton, Matthew-Simonton, and Creighton, 62.

83. Simonton, Matthew-Simonton, and Creighton, 87.

84. Simonton, Matthew-Simonton, and Creighton, 77.

85. Simonton, Matthew-Simonton, and Creighton, 72, 73.

86. Currell, 48.

87. Currell, 47.

88. Bernie S. Siegel, *Love, Medicine, and Miracles: Lessons Learned about Self-Healing from a Surgeon's Experience with Exceptional Patients* (New York: Harper and Row, 1986), 18.

89. Siegel, *Love, Medicine, and Miracles* 21.

90. Siegel, 75.

91. Siegel, 78.

92. Siegel, 84–85.

93. Siegel, 94.

94. Siegel, 223, 26.

95. Siegel, 23.

96. Siegel, 94.

97. Snyder and Mitchell, 44–45.

98. Snyder and Mitchell, 44.

99. Arthur J. Barsky, *Worried Sick: Our Troubled Quest for Wellness* (Boston: Little Brown, 1988), 145.

100. Barsky, *Worried Sick*, 145.

101. Barsky, 145.

102. Martin E. P. Seligman and Mihaly Csikszentmihalyi, "Positive Psychology: An Introduction," *American Psychologist* 55, no. 1 (2000): 5.

103. Seligman and Csikszentmihalyi, "Positive Psychology," 10.

104. Seligman and Csikszentmihalyi, 10.

105. Barsky, 146.

106. LeShan, 133.

107. Ahmed, *Promise of Happiness*, 59.

108. Barbara S. Held, "The Tyranny of the Positive Attitude in America: Observation and Speculation," *Journal of Clinical Psychology* 58, no. 9 (2002): 956.

109. Erving Goffman, *The Presentation of Self in Everyday Life* (New York: Anchor Books, 1959), 56.

110. C. McGrath et al., "'Right' Way to 'Do' Illness? Thinking Critically about Positive Thinking," *Internal Medicine Journal* 36 (2006): 665.

111. Barrie R. Cassileth, "The Social Implications of Questionable Cancer Therapies," *CA: A Cancer Journal for Clinicians* 39, no. 5 (1989): 313.

112. Cassileth, "Social Implications," 315.

113. Cassileth, 315.

114. "Rehabilitation Can't Begin Too Soon," *Memorial Sloan-Kettering News*, April 3, 1978, folder 44, box 5, series 3, record group 375, Press Releases, MSKCC Library and Archives, RAC.

115. Ruth Shereff, "Wish Me Well," *Ms.*, October 1989, 26.

116. Shereff, "Wish Me Well," 26.

117. Shereff, 26.

118. Cassileth, 313.

119. Barbara Ehrenreich, *Natural Causes: An Epidemic of Wellness, the Certainty of Dying and Killing Ourselves to Live Longer* (New York: Hachette Book Group 2018), 64.

120. Azra Raza, *The First Cell and the Human Costs of Pursuing Cancer to the Last* (New York: Hachette Book Group, 2019), 7.

121. Elof Axel Carlson, "The Hoosier Connection: Compulsory Sterilization as Moral Hygiene," in *A Century of Eugenics in America: From the Indiana Experiment to the Human Genome Era*, ed. Paul A. Lombardo (Bloomington: Indiana University Press, 2011), 11.

122. Siegel, 26.

123. Snyder and Mitchell, 46.

124. Ahmed, 216.

125. Ahmed, 216.

Chapter 4

1. James T. Patterson, *The Dread Disease: Cancer and Modern American Culture* (Cambridge: Harvard University Press, 1987), 43.

2. Patterson, *Dread Disease*, 43–44.

3. Patterson, 60–61.

4. "Note on the Smoke Problem of Pittsburg in Its Relation to Cancer," Frederick L. Hoffman Papers, 1913–16, MS C 3 box 1 of 2, History of Medicine Division, National Library of Medicine.

5. "Note on the Smoke Problem of Pittsburg."

6. "Note on Cancer Statistics," Frederick L. Hoffman Papers, 1913–16, MS C 3 box 1 of 2, History of Medicine Division, National Library of Medicine.

7. "Cancer and Your Home," press release, ca. 1940, reel 1, vol. 1 (1939–49), series 4, subseries 3, record group 375, Public Affairs Scrapbooks, MSKCC Library and Archives, RAC.

8. John J. O'Neill, "Science: Diet to Prevent Cancer Sought: Doctors Study Added Clew to Chemical Cure: Experiments with Animal Believed Indicating Key, Big-Scale Test Planned," *New York Herald Tribune*, ca. 1940, reel 1, vol. 1 (1939–49), series 4, subseries 3, record group 375, Public Affairs Scrapbooks, MSKCC Library and Archives, RAC.

9. O'Neill, "Science: Diet to Prevent Cancer Sought."

10. *New York Herald Tribune*, ca. 1941; *Ladies Home Journal*, July 1941; "Cancer Related to Vitamin A Shortage," *Modern Science* 1941, scrapbook 5.2 (January 1941–March 1942), record group 375, Public Affairs Scrapbooks, MSKCC Library and Archives, RAC.

11. "Biotin May Promote Cancer (B Vitamin)," *Hospital Top Buy* (Chicago), 1942, scrapbook 5.2 (January 1941–March 1942), record group 375, Public Affairs Scrapbooks, MSKCC Library and Archives, RAC.

12. "Stomach Cancer More Prevalent among Japanese—Scientists Report Disease Occurs Two or Three Times as Frequently in Japs," *Niagara Falls Gazette* ([illegible month] 24, 1942), scrapbook 6: General Clippings (1942–44), series 4, subseries 3, record group 375, Public Affairs Scrapbooks, MSKCC Library and Archives, RAC.

13. "Formation of Cancer Prevention Committee Marks New Approach in Cancer Control," November 20, 1948, box 1 (1935–49), series 3, record group 375, Press Releases, MSKCC Library and Archives, RAC.

14. Patterson, 187.

15. "Announcement," 1958; press release, July 16, 1958; press release, July 12, 1958; folder 24 (1958), box 3 (1958–64), series 3, record group 375, Press Releases, MSKCC Library and Archives, RAC.

16. Press release, October 21, 1959, folder 25 (1959), box 3 (1958–64), series 3, record group 375, Press Releases, MSKCC Library and Archives, RAC.

17. Press release, October 20, 1959, folder 25 (1959), box 3 (1958–64), series 3, record group 375, Press Releases, MSKCC Library and Archives, RAC.

18. Press release, November 29, 1960, folder 26 (1960), box 3 (1958–64), series 3, record group 375, Press Releases, MSKCC Library and Archives, RAC.

19. Press release, November 29, 1960, folder 26 (1960), box 3 (1958–64), series 3, record group 375, Press Releases, MSKCC Library and Archives, RAC.

20. Press release, November 27, 1961, folder 27 (1961), box 3 (1958–64), series 3, record group 375, Press Releases, MSKCC Library and Archives, RAC.

21. Press release, February 15, 1961, folder 27 (1961); press release, April 14, 1962, folder 28 (1962), box 3 (1958–64), series 3, record group 375, Press Releases, MSKCC Library and Archives, RAC.

22. Press release, February 6, 1964, folder 30 (1964), box 3 (1958–64), series 3, record group 375, Press Releases, MSKCC Library and Archives, RAC.

23. Patterson, 61.

24. Patterson, 205–6.

25. Patterson, 208–11.

26. Patterson, 216–17.

27. Patterson, 256–57.

28. "The National Cancer Act: The Foundation of Cancer Research in the United States," Mary Lasker Papers, 1940–93, 1970 folder, box 79, series 111: Topical Files, Columbia University Rare Book and Manuscript Library.

29. "Sherman Fairchild Foundation Gives $4 Million to Memorial Sloan-Kettering," July 27, 1978, folder 44, box 5, series 3, record group 375, Press Releases, MSKCC Library and Archives, RAC.

30. "Some 40 Chemicals and Physical Agents . . . ," press release ca. 1978, folder 44, box 5, series 3, record group 375, Press Releases, MSKCC Library and Archives, RAC.

31. Patterson, 260; James S. Olson, *Making Cancer History: Disease and Discovery at the University of Texas M.D. Anderson Cancer Center* (Baltimore: Johns Hopkins University Press, 2009), 229.

32. Olson, *Making Cancer History*, 227.
33. Olson, *Making Cancer History*, 224.
34. Olson, *Making Cancer History*, 230.
35. S. Lachlann Jain, *Malignant: How Cancer Becomes Us* (Berkeley, University of California Press, 2013), 12.
36. "Science May Find Cancer Cure before the Cause," *Birmingham Post* (Birmingham, AL), July 20, 1942, scrapbook 6: General Clippings (1942–44), series 4, subseries 3, record group 375, Public Affairs Scrapbooks, MSKCC Library and Archives, RAC.
37. Frederick L. Hoffman, letter to Curtis E. Lakeman, November 16, 1915, Frederick L. Hoffman Papers, 1913–16, MS C 3 box 2 of 2, History of Medicine Division, National Library of Medicine.
38. Frederick L. Hoffman, letter to Curtis E. Lakeman, January 26, 1915, Frederick L. Hoffman Papers, 1913–16, MS C 3, box 2 of 2, History of Medicine Division, National Library of Medicine.
39. Frank Horsfall, letter of protest to John Heller, n.d., folder 36, box 2 (1961–69), series 6, record group 375, TV/Radio, MSKCC Library and Archives, RAC.
40. Richard G. Berger, "Prevent Cancer!" *Nature's Path*, October 1950, Mary Lasker Papers, 1940–93, folder 6 (1951), box 75, series 111: Topical Files, Columbia University Rare Book and Manuscript Library.
41. Berger, "Prevent Cancer."
42. Richard G. Berger, "Arrest Cancer, (Why Not?) It's Wanted for Murder!," ca. 1949, Mary Lasker Papers, 1940–93, folder 7 (1949), box 75, series 111: Topical Files, Columbia University Rare Book and Manuscript Library.
43. Richard G. Berger, column, *Nature's Path*, February 1951, Mary Lasker Papers, 1940–93, folder 6 (1951), box 75, series 111: Topical Files, Columbia University Rare Book and Manuscript Library.
44. "The Cure for Cancer Is Prevention," *California Farmer*, November 4, 1950, Mary Lasker Papers, 1940–93, folder 6 (1951), box 75, series 111: Topical Files, Columbia University Rare Book and Manuscript Library.
45. American Cancer Society, memo about cancer prevention, December 7, 1954, Mary Lasker Papers, 1940–93, folder 1 (1954), box 77, series 111: Topical Files, Columbia University Rare Book and Manuscript Library.
46. "Cure for Cancer Is Prevention."
47. Olson, *Making Cancer History*, 226.
48. Samuel S. Epstein, *The Politics of Cancer* (Garden City, NY: Anchor Books, 1978), 18.
49. Epstein, *Politics of Cancer*, 322.
50. Epstein, 343, xv.
51. Rose Kushner, *Breast Cancer: A Personal History and an Investigative Report* (New York: Harcourt Brace Jovanovich, 1975), 140.
52. Audre Lorde, *The Cancer Journals, Special Edition* (1980; repr., San Francisco: Aunt Lute Books, 1997), 61.
53. Lisa Diedrich, *Treatments: Language, Politics, and the Culture of Illness* (Minneapolis: University of Minnesota Press, 2007), 26.
54. Maren Klawiter, *The Biopolitics of Breast Cancer: Changing Cultures of Disease and Activism* (Minneapolis: University of Minnesota Press, 2008), 98; Diedrich, *Treatments*, 50.
55. Susan Rennie, "Breast Cancer Prevention: Diet vs. Drugs," *Ms.* 3, no. 6 (May/June 1993): 38.
56. Rennie, "Breast Cancer Prevention," 38.

57. Rennie, 38.

58. Liane Clorfene-Casten, "The Environmental Link to Breast Cancer," *Ms.* 3, no. 6 (May/June 1993): 52.

59. Clorfene-Castin, "Environmental Link," 54.

60. Liane Clorfene-Casten, "Inside the Cancer Establishment," *Ms.* 3, no. 6 (May/June 1993): 57.

61. Michele Landsberg, "Breast Cancer Conference: Clean the Earth, Save Lives," *Ms.* 8, no. 3 (November/December 1997): 17.

62. Patterson, 257.

63. Press release, October 19, 1959, folder 25 (1959), box 3 (1958–64), series 3, record group 375, Press Releases, MSKCC Library and Archives, RAC.

64. Klawiter, *Biopolitics of Breast Cancer*, 102.

65. Olson, *Making Cancer History*, 232–33.

66. Sharon L. Snyder and David T. Mitchell, *Cultural Locations of Disability* (Chicago: University of Chicago Press, 2006), 49.

67. Clarence C. Little, "Cancer Can Be Cured," ca. 1940, reel 1, vol. 1 (1939–41), record group 375, Public Affairs Scrapbooks, MSKCC Library and Archives, RAC.

68. Walter Ross, *Crusade: The Official History of the American Cancer Society* (New York: Arbor House, 1987), 183.

69. Ross, *Crusade*, 183–85.

70. Curtis E. Lakeman, "Cancer as a Social Problem," address to the National Conference of Charities and Correction, Memphis, TN, May 15, 1913, Frederick L. Hoffman Papers, 1913–16, MS C 3 box 1 of 2, History of Medicine Division, National Library of Medicine.

71. Lakeman, "Cancer as a Social Problem.".

72. Frederick L. Hoffman, "The Statistical Evidence of the Increase in Cancer," Frederick L. Hoffman Papers, 1913–16, MS C 3 box 1 of 2, History of Medicine Division, National Library of Medicine.

73. Lakeman, "Cancer as a Social Problem."

74. Frederick L. Hoffman, letter to Curtis E. Lakeman, April 1, 1914, Frederick L. Hoffman Papers, 1913–16, MS C 3, box 1 of 2, History of Medicine Division, National Library of Medicine.

75. "An Ounce of Prevention," *Reader's Digest*, October 1944, scrapbook 6: General Clippings (1942–44), series 4, subseries 3, record group 375, Public Affairs Scrapbooks, MSKCC Library and Archives, RAC.

76. *Endless Frontier*, script, radio program starring Raymond Massey, episode 2: "The Search," February 2, 1952, folder 2 (1952 radio programs), box 1, series 6, record group 375, Radio/TV Programs, MSKCC Library and Archives, RAC.

77. Little, "Cancer Can Be Cured."

78. Barbara Heimann, "Why I Don't Smoke," *American Cancer Society News*, 1965, Mary Lasker Papers, 1940–93, box 79, series 111: Topical Files, Columbia University Rare Book and Manuscript Library.

79. Edward Reynolds, "Cancer a Controllable Disease: How the Women's Clubs Can Help the Less Intelligent," June 24, 1915, address delivered at the Annual Meeting of the Massachusetts State Federation of Women's Clubs at Marion, Frederick L. Hoffman Papers, 1913–16, MS C 3, box 2 of 2, National Library of Medicine.

80. Reynolds, "Cancer a Controllable Disease."

81. US Department of Health, Education, and Welfare, Public Health Service, *End Results in Cancer, Report no. 2*, 1966, Mary Lasker Papers, 1940–93, box 79, series 111: Topical Files, Columbia University Rare Book and Manuscript Library.

82. Catherine E. Mosher and Sharon Danoff-Burg, "An Attributional Analysis of Gender and Cancer-Related Stigma," *Sex Roles* 59 (2008): 827.

83. Mosher and Danoff-Burg, "Attributional Analysis," 837.

84. "Formation of Cancer Prevention Committee Marks New Approach in Cancer Control," November 20, 1948, box 1 (1935–49), series 3, record group 375, Press Releases, MSKCC Library and Archives, RAC.

85. Susan Yadlon, "Skinny Women and Good Mothers: The Rhetoric of Risk, Control, and Culpability in the Production of Knowledge about Breast Cancer," *Feminist Studies* 23, no. 3 (Fall 1997): 646.

86. Yadlon, "Skinny Women and Good Mothers," 647, 648.

87. Zoltan Majdik and Carrie Anne Platt, "Selling Certainty: Genetic Complexity and Moral Urgency in Myriad Genetics' BRACAnalysis Campaign," *Rhetoric Society Quarterly* 42, no. 2 (2012): 122.

88. Majdik and Platt, "Selling Certainty," 122.

89. Majdik and Platt, 126–27.

90. Majdik and Platt, 131.

91. Epstein, *Politics of Cancer*, 492.

92. Epstein, 494.

93. Epstein, 494–95.

94. Karen Kopelson, "Risky Appeals: Recruiting to the Environmental Breast Cancer Movement in the Age of 'Pink Fatigue,'" *Rhetoric Society Quarterly*, 43 no. 2 (2013): 111–12.

95. Kopelson, "Risky Appeals," 119.

96. Kopelson, 121, 120.

97. Kopelson, 121.

98. Emilia Nielsen, *Disrupting Breast Cancer Narratives: Stories of Rage and Repair* (Toronto: University of Toronto Press, 2019), 86, 87.

99. Susan Sontag, *Illness as Metaphor and AIDS and Its Metaphors* (New York: Farrar, Straus, and Giroux, 1977), 40.

100. Emily E. Nye, "The Rhetoric of AIDS: A New Taxonomy," in *Embodied Rhetorics: Disability in Language and Culture*, ed. James C. Wilson and Cynthia Lewiecki-Wilson (Carbondale: Southern Illinois University Press, 2002), 237.

Chapter 5

1. "40 Times Trump Said the Coronavirus Would Go Away," *Washington Post*, November 2, 2020, online video.

2. Tamara Keith, "Trump Says He Prevented Panic on Pandemic. That's Not His Usual Approach," NPR, September 12, 2020, online.

3. Christine Sexton, "Coronavirus: Gov. DeSantis Wants Seniors and Seriously Ill People to Stay Home," *Daytona Beach News-Journal*, March 24, 2020, online.

4. Qtd. in Jay Dolmage, *Academic Ableism: Disability and Higher Education* (Ann Arbor: University of Michigan Press, 2017), 13.

5. Sharon L. Snyder and David T. Mitchell, *Cultural Locations of Disability* (Chicago: University of Chicago Press, 2006), 46.

6. Rosemarie Garland-Thomson, "Seeing the Disabled: Visual Rhetorics of Popular Photography," in *The New Disability History: American Perspectives*, ed. Paul K. Longmore and Lauri Umansky (New York: New York University Press, 2001), 348.

7. Judy Z. Segal, *Health and the Rhetoric of Medicine* (Carbondale: Southern Illinois University Press, 2005), 23.

8. Jay Dolmage, "Octalog III: The Politics of Historiography in 2010," ed. Lois Agnew, Laurie Gries, Zosha Stuckey, *Rhetoric Review* 30, no. 2 (2011): 113.

9. Dolmage, "Octalog III," 114.

10. Qtd. in Susan Wendell, "Unhealthy Disabled: Treating Chronic Illnesses as Disabilities," *The Disability Studies Reader*, ed. Lennard J. Davis (Mahwah, NJ: Routledge, 2013), 148.

11. Lennard Davis, *Enforcing Normalcy: Disability, Deafness, and the Body* (Brooklyn, NY: Verso, 1995), 140.

12. Curtis E. Lakeman, "Cancer as a Social Problem," address to the National Conference of Charities and Correction, Memphis, TN, May 15, 1913, Frederick L. Hoffman Papers, 1913–16, MS C 3 box 1 of 2, History of Medicine Division, National Library of Medicine.

13. S. Lochlann Jain, *Malignant: How Cancer Becomes Us* (Berkeley: University of California Press, 2013), 48.

14. Mary K. DeShazer, *Mammographies: The Cultural Discourse of Breast Cancer Narratives* (Ann Arbor: University of Michigan Press, 2013), 9.

15. Samantha King, "Pink Ribbons Inc.: Breast Cancer Activism and the Politics of Philanthropy," *International Journal of Qualitative Studies in Education*, 17, no. 4 (2004): 475, 489.

16. Kate Pickert, *Radical: The Science, Culture, and History of Breast Cancer in America* (Boston: Little, Brown, Spark, 2019), 251.

17. Phaedra C. Pezzullo, "Resisting 'National Breast Cancer Awareness Month': The Rhetoric of Counterpublics and their Rhetorical Performance," *Quarterly Journal of Speech* 89, no. 4 (2003): 346.

18. Karen Kopelson, "Risky Appeals: Recruiting to the Environmental Breast Cancer Movement in the Age of 'Pink Fatigue,'" *Rhetoric Society Quarterly* 43, no. 2 (2013): 108.

19. Gayle A. Sulik, *Pink Ribbon Blues: How Breast Cancer Culture Undermines Women's Health* (New York: Oxford University Press, 2011), 9.

20. Lennard J. Davis, "Bodies of Difference: Politics, Disability, and Representation," in *Disability Studies: Enabling the Humanities*, ed. Sharon L. Snyder, Brenda Jo Brueggemann, and Rosemarie Garland Thomson (New York: Modern Language Association, 2002), 106.

21. Jain, *Malignant*, 199.

22. Audre Lorde, *The Cancer Journals, Special Edition*, 1980 (San Francisco: Aunt Lute Books, 1987), 42.

23. Lorde, *Cancer Journals*, 41–42.

24. Dolmage, "Octalog III," 114.

25. Lisa Diedrich, *Treatments: Language, Politics, and the Culture of Illness* (Minneapolis: University of Minnesota Press, 2007), 26, 50.

26. Lorde, 42.

27. Emilia Nielsen, *Disrupting Breast Cancer Narratives: Stories of Rage and Repair* (Toronto: University of Toronto, 2019), 5.

28. Lorde, 42.

29. Lorde, 61.

30. Eli Clare, *Brilliant Imperfection: Grappling with Cure* (Durham, NC: Duke University Press, 2017), 41.

31. Diedrich, *Treatments*, 54, 61.

32. Diedrich, 46.

33. Lorde, 20.

34. Clare, *Brilliant Imperfection*, 87.

35. Christa Teston, *Bodies in Flux: Scientific Methods for Negotiating Medical Uncertainty* (Chicago: University of Chicago Press, 2017), 176.

36. Jain, 219.

37. Leah Lakshmi Piepzna-Samarasinha, *Care Work: Dreaming Disability Justice* (Vancouver: Arsenal Pulp Press, 2018), chap. 1, E-book.

38. Virginia Held, "Care Ethics and the Social Contract," in *The Ethics of Care: The State of the Art*, ed. Frans Vosman, Andries Baart, and Jaco Hoffman (Leuven: Peeters Publishers, 2020), 149.

39. A. Suresh Canagarajah, *Language Incompetence: Learning to Communicate through Cancer, Disability, and Anomalous Embodiment* (New York: Routledge, 2022), 23, E-book.

40. Canagarajah, *Language Incompetence*, 50.

41. Alice Wong, "I'm Disabled and Need a Ventilator to Live. Am I Expendable during This Pandemic?" *Vox*, April 4, 2020, online.

42. Susan Wendell, "Unhealthy Disabled: Treating Chronic Illnesses as Disabilities," in Davis, *Disability Studies Reader*, 171.

43. Wendell, "Unhealthy Disabled," 171.

44. Jessica Restaino, *Surrender: Feminist Rhetoric and Ethics in Love and Illness* (Carbondale: Southern Illinois University Press, 2019), 14.

45. Galton, qtd. in Dolmage, *Academic Ableism*, 13

46. Sara Ahmed, *The Promise of Happiness* (Durham, NC: Duke University Press, 2010), 216.

WORKS CITED

Archival Material

Historical Resources Center, Research Medical Library, University of Texas MD Anderson Cancer Center, Houston, TX.

Mary Lasker Papers (1940–93). Rare Book and Manuscript Library, Columbia University in the City of New York.

Frederick L. Hoffman Papers (1913–16). History of Medicine Division, National Library of Medicine, National Institutes of Health, Bethesda, MD.

Memorial Sloan Kettering Cancer Center Library and Archives (MSKCC), Rockefeller Archive Center (RAC), Sleepy Hollow, New York.

Published Sources

Ahmed, Sara. *The Promise of Happiness.* Durham, NC: Duke University Press, 2010.

Annas, George J. "Reframing the Debate on Health Care: Reform by Replacing Our Metaphors." *New England Journal of Medicine* 332, no. 11 (1995): 744–47.

Arney, Kat. "Podcast: The Dark Connection between Cancer Research and the Eugenics Movement." Genetic Literacy Project: Science Not Ideology. Online.

Barsky, Arthur J., MD. *Worried Sick: Our Troubled Quest for Wellness.* Boston: Little, Brown, 1988.

Bashford, Alison, and Philippa Levine, eds. *The Oxford Handbook of the History of Eugenics.* New York: Oxford University Press, 2010.

Baynton, Douglas C. "Disability and the Justification of Inequality in American History." In Longmore and Umansky, *New Disability History,* 33–57.

Birke, Lynda. "Bodies and Biology." In *Feminist Theory and the Body,* edited by Janet Price and Margrit Shildrick, 42–49. Mahwah, NJ: Routledge, 1999.

Braun, Michael. "Classics in Oncology: Portrait of Arthur M. Sutherland, MD." *CA-A Cancer Journal for Clinicians* 31, no. 3 (May/June 1981): 156–58.

Burke, Kenneth. *Permanence and Change.* Berkeley: University of California Press, 1954.

Byrom, Brad. "A Pupil and a Patient: Hospital Schools in Progressive America." In Longmore and Umansky, *New Disability History,* 133–56.

Canagarajah, A. Suresh. *Language Incompetence: Learning to Communicate through Cancer, Disability, and Anomalous Embodiment.* New York: Routledge, 2022. E-book.

"Cancer-Fighter Cornelius P. Rhoads: Some Gangsters Are Vulnerable." *Time,* June 27, 1949. Online.

Carlson, Elof Axel. "The Hoosier Connection: Compulsory Sterilization as Moral Hygiene." In Lombardo, *A Century of Eugenics in America,* 11–25.

Cassileth, Barrie R. "The Social Implications of Questionable Cancer Therapies." *CA: A Cancer Journal for Clinicians* 39, no. 5 (1989): 311–16.

Ceccarelli, Leah. *On the Frontier of Science: An American Rhetoric of Exploration and Exploitation.* East Lansing: Michigan State University Press, 2013.

Childe, Charles P. *The Control of a Scourge, or How Cancer Is Curable.* New York: E. P. Dutton, 1907.

Clare, Eli. *Brilliant Imperfection: Grappling with Cure*. Durham, NC: Duke University Press, 2017.

Clorfene-Casten, Liane. "The Environmental Link to Breast Cancer." *Ms.* 3, no. 6 (May/June 1962): 52–56.

———. "Inside the Cancer Establishment." *Ms.* 3, no. 6 (May/June 1993): 57.

Crook, Tom. *Governing Systems: Modernity and the Making of Public Health in England, 1830–1910*. Berkeley Series in British Studies. Vol. 11. Berkeley: University of California Press, 2016.

Currell, Susan. "Eugenic Decline and Recovery in Self-Improvement Literature of the Thirties." In Currell and Cogdell, *Popular Eugenics*, 44–69.

Currell, Susan, and Christina Cogdell. "Introduction." In Currell and Cogdell, *Popular Eugenics*, 1–14.

Currell, Susan, and Christina Cogdell, eds. *Popular Eugenics: National Efficiency and American Mass Culture in the 1930s*. Athens: Ohio University Press, 2006.

Davis, Lennard J. "Bodies of Difference: Politics, Disability, and Representation." In *Disability Studies: Enabling the Humanities*, edited by Sharon L. Snyder, Brenda Jo Brueggemann, and Rosemarie Garland-Thomson, 100–106. New York: Modern Language Association, 2002.

———. *Enforcing Normalcy: Disability, Deafness, and the Body*. Brooklyn: Verso, 1995.

DeShazer, Mary K. *Mammographies: The Cultural Discourses of Breast Cancer Narratives*. Ann Arbor: University of Michigan Press, 2013.

Diedrich, Lisa. *Treatments: Language, Politics, and the Culture of Illness*. Minneapolis: University of Minnesota Press, 2007.

Dolmage, Jay Timothy. *Academic Ableism: Disability and Higher Education*. Ann Arbor: University of Michigan Press, 2017.

———. "Disability Rhetorics." In *The Cambridge Companion to Literature and Disability*, edited by Clare Barker and Stuart Murray, 212–26. Cambridge, UK: Cambridge University Press, 2017.

———. *Disability Rhetoric*. Syracuse, NY: Syracuse University Press, 2014.

———. "Octalog III: The Politics of Historiography in 2010." Edited by Lois Agnew, Laurie Gries, and Zosha Stuckey. Coauthored with Vicki Tolar Burton, Jay Dolmage, Jessica Enoch, Ronald L. Jackson II, LuMing Mao, Malea Powell, Arthur E. Walzer, Ralph Cintron, and Victor Vitanza. *Rhetoric Review* 30, no. 2 (2011): 109–34.

Dubriwny, Tasha N. *The Vulnerable Empowered Woman: Feminism, Postfeminism, and Women's Health*. New Brunswick, NJ: Rutgers University Press, 2012.

Ehrenreich, Barbara. *Bright-Sided: How the Relentless Promotion of Positive Thinking has Undermined America*. New York: Metropolitan Books, 2009.

———. *Natural Causes: An Epidemic of Wellness, the Certainty of Dying and Killing Ourselves to Live Longer*. New York: Hachette Book Group, 2018.

Epstein, Samuel S. *The Politics of Cancer*. Garden City, NY: Anchor Books, 1978.

Erevelles, Nirmala. *Disability and Difference in Global Contexts: Enabling a Transformative Body Politic*. London: Palgrave Macmillan, 2011.

Evans, Richard I. *Dialogue with C. G. Jung*. Dialogues in Contemporary Psychology Series. New York: Praeger, 1981.

Fahnestock, Jeanne. *Rhetorical Figures in Science*. New York: Oxford University Press, 1999.

"40 Times Trump Said the Coronavirus Would Go Away." *Washington Post*, November 2, 2020. Online video.

Foss, Sonja K. *Rhetorical Criticism: Exploration and Practice*. 4th ed. Long Grove, IL: Waveland, 2009.

Gardner, Kirsten E. *Early Detection: Women, Cancer, and Awareness Campaigns in the Twentieth-Century United States.* Chapel Hill: University of North Carolina Press, 2006.

Garland-Thomson, Rosemarie. *Extraordinary Bodies: Figuring Physical Disability in American Culture and Literature.* Columbia University Press, 1997.

———. "Seeing the Disabled: Visual Rhetorics of Popular Photography." In Longmore and Umansky, *New Disability History*, 335–74.

Garrison, Kristen. "The Personal Is Rhetorical: War, Protest, and Peace in Breast Cancer Narratives." *Disability Studies Quarterly* 27, no. 4 (2004).

Glenn, Cheryl. *Unspoken: A Rhetoric of Silence.* Carbondale: Southern Illinois University Press, 2004.

Goffman, Erving. *The Presentation of Self in Everyday Life.* New York: Anchor, 1959.

———. *Stigma: Notes on the Management of Spoiled Identity.* Hoboken, NJ: Prentice-Hall, 1963.

Graves, Liz. "Auditorium Honoring Jackson Laboratory Founder C. C. Little to be Renamed." *Mount Desert Islander*, September 20, 2021. Online.

Held, Barbara S. "The Tyranny of the Positive Attitude in America: Observation and Speculation." *Journal of Clinical Psychology* 58, no. 9 (2002): 965–92.

Held, Virginia. "Care Ethics and the Social Contract." In *The Ethics of Care: The State of the Art*, edited by Frans Vosman, Andries Baart, Jaco Hoffman, 137–62. Leuven: Peeters Publishers, 2020.

Hickel, K. Walter. "Medicine, Bureaucracy, and Social Welfare: The Politics of Disability Compensation for American Veterans of World War I." In Longmore and Umansky, *New Disability History*, 236–67.

Jain, S. Lochlann. *Malignant: How Cancer Becomes Us.* Berkeley: University of California Press, 2013.

Keith, Tamara. "Trump Says He Prevented Panic on Pandemic. That's Not His Usual Approach." NPR, September 12, 2020. Online.

Keränen, Lisa. *Scientific Characters: Rhetoric, Politics, and Trust in Breast Cancer Research.* Tuscaloosa: University of Alabama Press, 2010.

King, Samantha. "Pink Ribbons Inc: Breast Cancer Activism and the Politics of Philanthropy." *International Journal of Qualitative Studies in Education* 17, no. 4 (2004): 473–92. Online.

Klawiter, Maren. *The Biopolitics of Breast Cancer: Changing Cultures of Disease and Activism.* Minneapolis: University of Minnesota Press, 2008.

Kline, Wendy. "Eugenics in the United States." In Bashford and Levine, *Oxford Handbook of the History of Eugenics*, 511–22.

Kopelson, Karen. "Risky Appeals: Recruiting to the Environmental Breast Cancer Movement in the Age of 'Pink Fatigue.'" *Rhetoric Society Quarterly* 43, no. 2 (2013): 107–33.

Kushner, Rose. *Breast Cancer: A Personal History and an Investigative Report.* New York: Harcourt Brace Jovanovich, 1975.

Lakoff, George, and Mark Johnson. *Metaphors We Live By.* Chicago: University of Chicago Press, 1980.

Landsberg, Michele. "Breast Cancer Conference: Clean the Earth, Save Lives." *Ms.* 8, no. 3 (November/December 1997): 12–17.

LeShan, Lawrence. *You Can Fight for Your Life: Emotional Factors in the Treatment of Cancer.* Foreword by Carl Simonton. New York: M. Evans, 1977.

Lindgren, Kristen. "Bodies in Trouble: Identity, Embodiment, and Disability." In *Gendering Disability*, edited by Bonnie G. Smith and Beth Hutchison, 145–65. New Brunswick, NJ: Rutgers University Press, 2004.

Linton, Simi. "What Is Disability Studies?" *PMLA* 120, no. 2 (2005): 518–22.

Lombardo, Paul A. "Introduction: Looking Back at Eugenics." In Lombardo, *A Century of Eugenics in America,* 1–8.

Lombardo, Paul A., ed. *A Century of Eugenics in America.* Bloomington: University of Indiana Press, 2011.

Longmore, Paul K. and Lauri Umanski, eds. *The New Disability History: American Perspectives.* New York: New York University Press, 2001.

Lorde, Audre. *The Cancer Journals, Special Edition.* 1980. Repr., San Francisco: Aunt Lute Books, 1997.

Love, Lauren. "U-M to Remove Little, Winchell Names from Campus Facilities." *University Record,* University of Michigan, March 29, 2018. Online.

Majdik, Zoltan, and Carrie Anne Platt. "Selling Certainty: Genetic Complexity and Moral Urgency in Myriad Genetics' BRACAnalysis Campaign." *Rhetoric Society Quarterly* 42, no. 2 (2012): 120–43.

McGee, Michael C. "In Search of 'The People': A Rhetorical Alternative." *Quarterly Journal of Speech* 61, no. 3 (1975): 235–49.

McGrath, C., C. F. C. Jordens, K. Montgomery, and I. H. Kerridge. "'Right' Way to 'Do' Illness? Thinking Critically about Positive Thinking." *Internal Medicine Journal* 36 (2006): 665–68.

Miller, Carolyn. "The Presumptions of Expertise: The Role of Ethos in Risk Analysis." *Configurations* 11, no. 2 (2003): 163–202.

Mitchell, David T., with Sharon L. Snyder. *The Biopolitics of Disability: Neoliberalism, Ablenationalism, and Peripheral Embodiment.* Ann Arbor: University of Michigan Press, 2015.

Mol, Annemarie. *The Body Multiple: Ontology in Medical Practice.* Durham, NC: Duke University Press, 2003.

Mosher, Catherine E., and Sharon Danoff-Burg. "An Attributional Analysis of Gender and Cancer-Related Stigma." *Sex Roles* 59 (2008): 827–38.

Mukherjee, Siddhartha. *The Emperor of All Maladies: A Biography of Cancer.* New York: Scribner, 2010.

Nielsen, Emilia. *Disrupting Breast Cancer Narratives: Stories of Rage and Repair.* Toronto: University of Toronto Press, 2019.

Nye, Emily E. "The Rhetoric of AIDS: A New Taxonomy." In *Embodied Rhetorics: Disability in Language and Culture,* edited by James C. Wilson and Cynthia Lewiecki-Wilson, 229–43. Carbondale: Southern Illinois University Press, 2002.

Olson, James S. *Bathsheba's Breast: Women, Cancer, and History.* Baltimore: Johns Hopkins University Press, 2002.

———. *Making Cancer History: Disease and Discovery at the University of Texas M.D. Anderson Cancer Center.* Baltimore: Johns Hopkins University Press, 2009.

Patterson, James T. *The Dread Disease: Cancer and Modern American Culture.* Cambridge, MA: Harvard University Press, 1987.

Paul, Diane B., and James Moore. "The Darwinian Context: Evolution and Inheritance." In *Oxford Handbook of the History of Eugenics,* edited by Alison Bashford and Philippa Levine, 27-42.

Pezzullo, Phaedra C. "Resisting 'National Breast Cancer Awareness Month': The Rhetoric of Counterpublics and Their Rhetorical Performance." *Quarterly Journal of Speech* 89, no. 4 (2003): 345–65.

Pickert, Kate. *Radical: The Science, Culture, and History of Breast Cancer in America.* Boston: Little, Brown Spark, 2019.

Piepzna-Samarasinha, Leah Lakshmi. *Care Work: Dreaming Disability Justice*. Vancouver: Arsenal Pulp Press, 2018. E-book.

Raza, Azra. *The First Cell and the Human Costs of Pursuing Cancer to the Last*. New York: Hachette, 2019.

Rennie, Susan. "Breast Cancer Prevention: Diet vs. Drugs." *Ms.* 3, no. 6 (May/June 1993).

Restaino, Jessica. *Surrender: Feminist Rhetoric and Ethics in Love and Illness*. Carbondale: Southern Illinois University Press, 2019.

Ross, Walter. *Crusade: The Official History of the American Cancer Society*. New York: Arbor House, 1987.

Rydell, Robert W. *World of Fairs: The Century-of-Progress Expositions*. Chicago: University of Chicago Press, 1993.

Sarewitz, Daniel. "Saving Science." *New Atlantis: A Journal of Technology and Society*, Spring/Summer 2016. Online.

Segal, Judy Z. "Breast Cancer Narratives as Public Rhetoric: Genre Itself and the Maintenance of Ignorance." *Linguistics and the Human Sciences* 3, no. 1 (2007): 3–23.

———. *Health and the Rhetoric of Medicine*. Carbondale: Southern Illinois University Press, 2005.

———. "Public Discourse and Public Policy: Some Ways That Metaphor Constrains Health (Care)." *Journal of Medical Humanities* 18, no. 4 (1997): 217–31.

Seligman, Martin E. P., and Mihaly Csikszentmihalyi. "Positive Psychology: An Introduction." *American Psychologist* 55, no. 1 (2000): 5–14.

Sexton, Christine. "Coronavirus: Gov. DeSantis Wants Seniors and Seriously Ill People to Stay Home." *Daytona Beach News-Journal*, March 24, 2020. Online.

Shereff, Ruth. "Wish Me Well." *Ms.*, October 1989.

Siegel, Bernie S., MD. *Love, Medicine, and Miracles: Lessons Learned about Self-Healing from a Surgeon's Experience with Exceptional Patients*. New York: Harper and Row, 1986.

Simonton, O. Carl, MD, Stephanie Matthew-Simonton, and James Creighton. *Getting Well Again: A Step-by-Step, Self-Help Guide to Overcoming Cancer for Patients and Their Families*. New York: J. P. Tarcher, 1978.

Snyder, Sharon L., and David T. Mitchell. *Cultural Locations of Disability*. Chicago: University of Chicago Press, 2006.

Sontag, Susan. *Illness as Metaphor and AIDS and Its Metaphors*. New York: Farrar, Straus and Giroux, 1977.

Spiegel, Allen M. "The Jeremiah Metzger Lecture: A Brief History of Eugenics in America: Implications for Medicine in the 21st Century." Transactions of the American Clinical and Climatological Association 130 (2019): 216–34. US National Library of Medicine/National Institutes of Health. Online.

Stacey, Jackie. *Teratologies: A Cultural Study of Cancer*. Mahwah, NJ: Routledge, 1997.

Stiker, Henri-Jacques. *A History of Disability*. Translated by William Sayers. Ann Arbor: University of Michigan Press, 1999.

Sulik, Gayle A. *Pink Ribbon Blues: How Breast Cancer Culture Undermines Women's Health*. New York: Oxford University Press, 2011.

Teston, Christa. *Bodies in Flux: Scientific Methods for Negotiating Medical Uncertainty*. Chicago: University of Chicago Press, 2017.

Teucher, Ulrich. "The Therapeutic Psychopoetics of Cancer Metaphors: Challenges in Interdisciplinarity." *History of Intellectual Culture*, 3, no. 1 (2003): 1–15.

Wendell, Susan. "Unhealthy Disabled: Treating Chronic Illnesses as Disabilities." In *The Disability Studies Reader*, edited by Lennard J. Davis, 161–73. Mahwah, NJ: Routledge, 2013.

Williams-Searle, John. "Cold Charity: Manhood, Brotherhood, and the Transformation of Disability, 1870–1900." In Longmore and Umansky, *New Disability History*.

Wong, Alice. "I'm Disabled and Need a Ventilator to Live. Am I Expendable during This Pandemic?" *Vox*, April 4, 2020. Online.

Woodstock, Louise. "Think about It: The Misbegotten Promise of Positive Thinking Discourse." *Journal of Communication Inquiry* 31, no. 2 (2007): 166–89.

Yadlon, Susan. "Skinny Women and Good Mothers: The Rhetoric of Risk, Control, and Culpability in the Production of Knowledge about Breast Cancer." *Feminist Studies* 23, no. 3 (Fall 1997): 645–77.

Ziege, Eva-Marie. "Patterns within Prejudice: Antisemitism in the United States in the 1940s." *Patterns of Prejudice* 46, no. 2 (2012): 93–127.

INDEX